OXFORD MEDICAL PUBLICATIONS

ASSISTING THE ANAESTHETIST

ASSISTING
THE ANAESTHETIST

Edited by

N. S. Morton

Consultant in Paediatric Anaesthesia & Intensive Care,
Royal Hospital for Sick Children, Glasgow

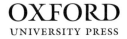

NHS

Institute for Innovation and Improvement

National Library for Health

www.library.nhs.uk
0800 555 550

"From knowledge to health"

OXFORD
UNIVERSITY PRESS

OXFORD
UNIVERSITY PRESS

Great Clarendon Street, Oxford OX2 6DP

Oxford University Press is a department of the University of Oxford.
It furthers the University's objective of excellence in research, scholarship,
and education by publishing worldwide in

Oxford New York

Athens Auckland Bangkok Bogotá Buenos Aires Calcutta
Cape Town Chennai Dar es Salaam Delhi Florence Hong Kong Istanbul
Karachi Kuala Lumpur Madrid Melbourne Mexico City Mumbai
Nairobi Paris São Paulo Singapore Taipei Tokyo Toronto Warsaw

with associated companies in Berlin Ibadan

Oxford is a registered trade mark of Oxford University Press
in the UK and in certain other countries

Published in the United States
by Oxford University Press Inc., New York

© N. S. Morton, 1997

First published 1997
Reprinted 2000, 2001

A catalogue record for this book is available from the British Library

Library of Congress Cataloging in Publication Data
(Data available)
ISBN 0 19 262444 X (Hbk)
ISBN 0 19 262443 1 (Pbk)

Printed in Great Britain
on acid-free paper by
Bookcraft (Bath) Ltd., Midsomer Norton, Avon

PREFACE

The trained assistant is essential for the safe conduct of modern anaesthesia. Vocational training courses for anaesthetic assistants have been developed which have national recognition in the United Kingdom. Local courses also occur and can be very good, although often they are not comprehensive and are not practically orientated. For national and local courses, the information which trainees need is scattered throughout many anaesthetic and nursing textbooks and is often written in too detailed and technical language. This book aims to bring together the essential information for the anaesthetic assistant into one text, to simplify and explain the jargon and to guide the reader to more detailed sources of further knowledge. The curriculum for the anaesthetic modules of the NVQ/SVQ Level 3 qualification is covered. There is no substitute for one-to-one clinical teaching but I hope this textbook will clarify and explain the most important aspects of assisting the anaesthetist.

Neil S. Morton.
April, 1997.
Glasgow.

ACKNOWLEDGEMENTS

I would like to thank all the contributors for their concise and practical chapters.

CONTENTS

SECTION 6   ANAESTHESIA FOR SPECIALTY SURGERY

List of Contributors

J. H. BROWN
Consultant Anaesthetist, Western Infirmary, Glasgow

W. DAVIS
Principal Physicist, Department of Anaesthesia, Western Infirmary, Glasgow

G. GILLIES
Consultant Anaesthetist, Victoria Infirmary, Glasgow

E. HOLMES
Clinical Nurse Tutor, School of Nursing, Southern General Hospital, Glasgow

H. HOSIE
Consultant Anaesthetist, Southern General Hospital, Glasgow

T. D. McCUBBIN
Consultant Anaesthetist, Western Infirmary, Glasgow

M. McNEIL
Consultant Anaesthetist, Royal Infirmary, Glasgow

N. S. MORTON
Consultant in Paediatric Anaesthesia and Intensive Care, Department of Anaesthesia, Royal Hospital for Sick Children, Glasgow

D. PAUL
Consultant Anaesthetist, Royal Infirmary, Glasgow

K. M. ROGERS
Consultant Anaesthetist, Western Infirmary, Glasgow

C. J. RUNCIE
Consultant Anaesthetist, Western Infirmary, Glasgow

D. WALKER
Consultant Anaesthetist, Southern General Hospital, Glasgow

SECTION 1

PREPARATION FOR ANAESTHESIA AND SURGERY

1. Preparation of the Patient and Preoperative Checks

H. Hosie, E. Holmes

Preoperative Checks

The ward staff start preparing the patient for anaesthesia and surgery by assessing the patient. Theatre staff continue this process but also take on the responsibilities of caring for a patient whose judgement may be impaired due to premedicant drugs or who may be unconscious. The role of the anaesthetic assistant includes acting as the patient's advocate, protecting the patient's dignity and rights, and ensuring that the correct procedures are adhered to. Many units have designed a checklist to record the preparation of the patient (an example is shown below). Unfortunately, most checklists are based on physical measurements and assessments and may have little or no space to document the psychological preparation or effects of premedication on the patient, although this is of great importance.

Identity

This is the single most vital check to be made. Is the patient arriving in the anaesthetic room the one you expect? The identity of the patient is confirmed by the ward nurses and the theatre personnel receiving the patient by:

1. checking verbally with the patient,
2. checking visually with the notes,
3. checking the patient's identity bracelet.

Remember that a premedicated patient may be unable to reliably recall events after premedication has had its effect. Where possible confirm all details with a third party such as the nurse escort. This policy is particularly important in children, the mentally handicapped and the unconscious patient, where details should be confirmed with parents, guardians and carers where appropriate.

Procedure

Omission of this check is one of the most common causes for litigation in the United Kingdom. The operation should be entered on the checklist, and should correspond with that on the operation slip, operating list, consent form and clinical notes.

Consent

Check the consent form with the patient and the ward nurse – any discrepancies must be brought to the attention of the anaesthetist and the surgeon performing the operation BEFORE anaesthesia is induced.

Ensure that the consent form is signed by the patient or a person who is legally responsible for a child, mentally handicapped patient or unconscious patient. This may be a parent or a legal guardian such as a social worker, director of a nursing home or a carer.

It is the patient's right to give or withhold consent, provided they understand the implications of their decision and have enough information to go on (except in certain situations under The Mental Health Act).

What information should be given preoperatively? Many health authorities, trusts and hospitals are reviewing their consent procedures and modifying the operation consent forms to ensure the patients are given sufficient information before signing the consent form. Patients can sign the consent form if they are capable of understanding the nature and consequences of the procedure and therefore children under the age of 16 may be able to sign their own consent forms. However, it is good practice to have the written consent of a parent or legal guardian as well. Patients have the right to refuse or to withdraw their consent at any time. Areas of particular concern involve young people under the age of 16 years, patients with language difficulties, patients with impaired sight, hearing or speech and patients with mental disorders.

There is also debate about what constitutes 'a procedure' which requires the patient's consent. For example, some units will ask labouring mothers to sign consent forms before giving epidural analgesia while in other units, verbal consent only is sought. Some patients may have invasive monitoring and analgesic infusions instituted without specific written consent being requested. Unit policy should be adhered to.

Consent should also be sought from patients who may be examined under anaesthesia by medical students or have procedures performed by non-medical personnel under medical direction. They may decide they do not wish to be examined or have students present. Again, unit policy should be adhered to.

Operation Site and Side

The operation site and side (right or left) should, if possible, be marked and be adequately prepared. The site should be verbally confirmed with the patient if possible and again the site should correspond to that entered on the consent form and operating list.

Preparation of the Skin

Units and individual surgeons vary in policies concerning preparation of the skin prior to surgery. Skin cleanliness is important to ensure the risk of wound infection is minimal. Research has shown that showering is better than bathing, but local policies vary. Chlorhexidine baths or treatment of the operation site with skin disinfectants are also used. Policies may vary with the type of operation, with more preparation when foreign material is being implanted, for example total joint replacement. Sometimes in life-saving emergency operations, only minimal skin preparation is possible.

Removal of hair from the operation site can be by shaving the site or by use of a depilatory cream. It is important that the site is not damaged by the razor or else infection rates may be high. In some units hair is removed after the patient is anaesthetized and you may be asked to do so. Recent research has suggested that the risk of infection is lowered when shaving is done at the time of operation.

Physiological Measurements

Most checklists will include recordings of the patient's weight, temperature, pulse, blood pressure and respiratory rate. A check on a sample of urine is made looking especially for sugar or blood. Weight is important in working out the correct dose of drugs, which are commonly given on a mg per kg basis, and is of particular importance when administering anaesthetic drugs to infants and children. The measurements give a baseline so that any abnormalities can be identified and corrected.

Test Results

Following the preoperative visits of the anaesthetist and surgeon, various investigations and tests may have been ordered. It is important that the results of these tests are available BEFORE anaesthesia is induced. It is distressing for everyone if a vital X-ray or test result has been lost or is not available and the operation is postponed or cancelled.

Allergies

Attention should be given to allergies, particularly to antibiotics or to skin cleansers, rubber, latex or adhesive tapes. All personnel should be reminded of these allergies.

Prosthetic Equipment

Under this salubrious title are items such as jewellery, hearing aids, false eyes, false limbs, wigs, spectacles and hairpins. Some units and some anaesthetists insist that all are removed before transfer to the anaesthetic room as such items are easily lost in the Bermuda triangle of the busy theatre suite! Some metallic objects may cause contact burns if surgical diathermy is used. However, removal of this type of personal item can provoke intense anxiety in some patients and removal of a hearing aid can impair communication markedly. The anaesthetist should be alerted to these personal items in a sensitive and appropriate way at a convenient moment. It is disconcerting, to say the least, to move a patient's head to prepare for intubation and find his hair comes off in your hand. Equally it is difficult to monitor depth of anaesthesia if you are looking at the pupil of a glass eye!

If patients do retain their prostheses during induction, but they are removed during the course of anaesthesia, it is essential that they are packed safely, labelled with the patient's name and unit number and kept with the patient's bed or trolley. Wedding rings may be taped to the patient's finger to ensure the ring is not lost during their stay in theatre.

Teeth and Dentures

Problems arising during anaesthesia involving teeth, crowns and bridgework account for a high proportion of legal cases against anaesthetists. The anaesthetist should check the location of dental work in any particular patient. It is a great help if an anaesthetic assistant reminds him of the presence of crowns and bridges.

The traditional attitude to the wearing of dentures is that they should be removed before the start of anaesthesia. A number of papers have suggested that the removal of dentures provokes extreme anxiety in many patients who fear loss of dignity and difficulty with communication. Methods of managing the airway have also changed, with the increasing use of the laryngeal mask and diminishing need for laryngoscopy and intubation. Many anaesthetists are now happy for patients to retain their dentures until induction of anaesthesia, with removal and safe storage thereafter.

Fasting

The fasting time is usually taught as a period of 6 hours to ensure complete emptying of the stomach thus preventing the danger of stomach acid coming up into the patient's airway. Studies have shown that, in some patients, particularly those in pain, after an injury or those given opiates, the stomach may not be empty even after this period of fasting. Recent studies suggest that, in patients with normal gastric emptying, clear fluids (not including any fat such as milk) can be safely taken for up to two hours before surgery with no risk of causing large volumes of acid gastric contents. Anaesthetic departments vary considerable in their policies for preoperative fasting and you may find individual anaesthetists also vary.

An easily remembered guideline is 6 – 4 – 3, that is 6 hours for solids (including milk or milky drinks), 4 hours for breast fed infants, and 3 hours for clear fluids (including water, juice, tea and coffee). Emergency cases should always be assumed to have a full stomach.

Other Checks

Check that the patient has voided urine and their bowels have moved. This is to prevent embarrassment to the patient and may be essential for some forms of surgery. Some patients may have a stoma (where the bowel is brought out at the skin surface to empty into a bag) and it is important to let theatre staff know this as they will need extra equipment for skin preparation. The patient may also have a urinary catheter, chest drain, nasogastric tube, feeding line or monitoring lines all in situ. All of these need specific care during transfer and surgery and sufficient trained personnel will need to be available to move and position the patient safely.

You may find the ward staff have recorded the patients response to the premedication. If not, make your own assessment of how the patient is (drowsy, deeply asleep, alert, anxious, terrified) and care for the patient accordingly. Continuous observation, information and reassurance is essential. The patient must NEVER be left alone once received into the theatre suite.

You may have to be aware of the patient's religious practices to care for the patient as a whole person. For instance, Jehovah's Witnesses may refuse transfusion of blood products.

All members of the theatre team contribute to the care planned by the ward staff by ensuring that the physical, spiritual and psychological aspects of care are continued. It is important that each patient is treated as an individual with respect and dignity and that all information about patients is kept confidential.

PREOPERATIVE VISITING

All patients should be visited by the surgeon and the anaesthetist or their deputies before the operation. The surgeon discusses the operation and its effects and obtains consent for surgery. The anaesthetist visits the patient to ensure they are in the best possible physical and mental condition for anaesthesia and surgery. They do this by introducing themselves to the patient, telling the patient what to expect and answering their questions and worries and discussing proposed anaesthetic and pain relief techniques. Consent is sought for invasive procedures and the medical condition of the patient is assessed by means of history, examination and investigations. This aspect of preoperative preparation is very important. Ward and theatre staff can help by reinforcing the information given, assessing the patient's mental and physical well-being and allaying anxiety.

Whereas the hospital world is familiar to us, remember that often to the patient, everything is very strange and frightening. They don't know the routines, are unfamiliar with the uniforms and different professionals they meet during their stay and are trusting strangers to look after them while they are unconscious and defenceless. Little wonder then that what to us is minor, everyday and routine becomes major, unusual and terrifying to the patient. Many find the loss of control very upsetting and disorientating.

Taking time to remember that every patient is a human being with fears, worries and rights just like yourself is essential. It is very important to introduce yourself to the patient, and explain even the most everyday of procedures. Above all, remember to behave in a professional manner and **treat every patient as you would wish to be treated yourself.**

At the preoperative visit, the anaesthetist will often give the patient an approximate time for surgery. They may tell them about transfer arrangements and about monitoring in the anaesthetic room. They will probably discuss the induction of anaesthesia and the wakening period in the recovery area. They usually discuss pain relief techniques and discuss the problem of sickness after surgery. Patients, however, often forget what they are told and it is important that ward and theatre staff reinforce these messages. Remember too that some patients will wish to deny their illness and distance themselves from it by adopting a passive role and 'putting themselves in your hands'. Others do not wish to know the details of their care as long as they get better.

The anaesthetist discuss premedication with the patient. In some regions theatre personnel are engaged in visiting patients before and after surgery. This allows theatre staff to assess the patient as a whole person. It also allows theatre staff to plan the care the patient will receive and afterwards evaluate how effective it has been. The visit allows the theatre staff to answer questions and reinforce information already given to the patient.

The patient may ask for more information about their operation or disease. They may also express fears about the anaesthetic. Please do not be tempted to speculate as this may cause distress to the patient, especially if there is a difference between what you have said and what someone else has said. It may reduce confidence and trust and produce an irate anaesthetist or surgeon. Try to answer what you do know, for example transfer to theatre, checking of patient details, anaesthetic room procedure and postoperative care (including frequent measurement of blood pressure, temperature, pulse oximetry, oxygen administration, intravenous infusions, blood transfusions, pain relief, wound drainage and wound dressings).

Optimal care can be achieved if the anaesthetist and his assistant are able to work together as a team in planning the anaesthetic management of a surgical list. The best scenario would be that the team meet following the anaesthetist's preoperative visit to discuss the management of individual patients (including special techniques and equipment) and that the patient is then revisited by the anaesthetic assistant. It is ideal if this continuity can be extended into the period after surgery.

Patients admitted for day surgery present particular problems. There is little time to establish rapport and, because they are to go home later the same day, premedication is not usually given. It is good practice for the anaesthetist and surgeon to do a round of the patients before the list starts and the anaesthetic assistant can take part in this round.

Patients admitted for emergency surgery present different management problems. The decision to take the patient to theatre is taken relatively quickly and less time is available to communicate with the patient. They will already be stressed and anxious following emergency admission, will have little time to acclimatize themselves to the ward or to the people caring for them and are psychologically unprepared. The needs of these patients are the same if not greater than routine elective cases. They need careful unhurried care, explanation and reassurance.

ASSESSMENT OF FITNESS AND RISKS

The fitness of a patient for surgery will be assessed by the anaesthetist who will be giving the anaesthetic. This is firstly done by examining the junior doctor's clerking record or, in some day case units, examination of the responses recorded by nursing staff to specific questions. Relevant aspects of the history and examination are confirmed with the patient or by ordering or examining results of investigations before agreeing to induce anaesthesia.

It is important for patient, surgeon and anaesthetist to be aware of the risks associated with any operation. Patients who are at high risk may choose not to have the operation, surgeons may choose to perform a simpler, shorter procedure rather than a more radical alternative, and the anaesthetist may consult with colleagues or even refuse to anaesthetize certain high risk cases. An example might be a patient with severe heart disease who comes in for a cosmetic operation on their nose. Most would say the risks outweigh the benefits in such a case.

The most commonly used method of assessing the risk of death associated with anaesthesia and surgery is the ASA status (Table 1.1). ASA stands for American Society of Anesthesiologists and they devised the following system which grades patients from 1 to 5. They also include an E category which denotes emergency. Emergency surgery increases the risk of serious complications and of death no matter which ASA grade. No index or assessment is

Table 1.1

ASA CLASSIFICATION
ASA 1 A patient with no organic, physiological or biochemical disturbance; the pathological process for which operation is to be performed is localized and does not entail a systemic disturbance.
ASA 2 Mild to moderate systemic disturbance caused by either the condition to be treated surgically or by other pathophysiological processes.
ASA 3 Severe disturbance or disease from whatever cause, even though it may not be possible to define the degree of disability with finality.
ASA 4 Severe systemic disorders that are already life threatening not always correctable by operation.
ASA 5 The moribund patient who has little chance of survival but is submitted to operation in desperation.

100% accurate. Most patients but not all, assessed using the ASA status as grade 5 will die. Most, but not all, patients assessed as grade 1 will survive. Overall, it has been shown in studies, such as the Confidential Enquiry into Perioperative Deaths (CEPOD), that patients in the higher risk grades are more likely to die than patients who are ASA 1 or 2.

Other scoring systems are used for specific types of patient. For example, the Goldmann risk index is used to assess heart function in patients with heart disease who may present for surgery, but it is also limited in accuracy. Despite these reservations on the use of scoring systems or assessments, they serve to alert anaesthetic and surgical staff to those at highest risk, ensuring appropriate treatment by appropriate staff and at an appropriate time to ensure the best care and attention for those most seriously ill.

At the preoperative visit the anaesthetist will be particularly interested in the following areas. (Please note that for specific types of surgery and specific types of patients other questions and investigations may be relevant, and you are referred to Section 6 on Specialized Anaesthesia, Chapters 21–36.)

History

Past history of anaesthesia may be important. Anaesthetists generally ask patients if they have had any problems with anaesthetics previously or if anyone in their family has had a problem. Disorders such as inability to metabolize suxamethonium, muscle disease, malignant hyperthermia (see p. 159) and porphyria may be picked up from the history.

Some patients may have been sensitized to anaesthetic drugs and may report allergies either to specific drugs or to substances such as metal (present in staples) or rubber (in masks and gloves).

Some patients give a history of awareness with a past anaesthetic, which is a state where the patient can hear, feel and occasionally see what is going on whilst being unable to move because of muscle blockade produced by relaxant drugs. It is rare, but particularly associated with bronchoscopy and Caesarean section. Patients may be aware at intubation if the drug used to induce anaesthesia has worn off and there is some difficulty in intubation. They may also report a feeling like 'awareness' while in the recovery area if muscle relaxants are not adequately reversed. All these situations can be terrifying for the patient, who then dreads a repetition with subsequent anaesthetics. These patients must be identified and treated with candour and reassurance.

Between 30% and 50% of patients feel sick or are sick after anaesthesia. If patients say they are prone to sickness after anaesthesia and surgery or if they suffer from travel sickness, techniques avoiding opiates may be used or specific drugs may be given to prevent sickness (see p. 193).

Past Medical History

Usually the anaesthetist is interested in episodes of illness requiring hospitalization, but many patients do not volunteer important illnesses because they are chronic and part of their everyday life, for example diabetes, epilepsy, asthma, high blood pressure. A useful question is to ask about any medicines they are being given at present from their family doctor.

Specific Enquiry

The anaesthetist will check the case notes and will ask a range of questions designed to identify patients with problems with the various systems of the body. Most anaesthetists will concentrate on symptoms relating to the heart, circulation and lungs but may ask questions about other systems such as kidneys, liver, gut and brain. The aim is to quickly tease out the important points which will affect the anaesthetic technique and postoperative care.

Cardiovascular system

In the United Kingdom, heart disease is common. High blood pressure (hypertension) is one sign of heart disease and patients with hypertension which is not controlled run a greater risk during anaesthesia and surgery compared with those with a normal blood pressure. Blood pressure should be stabilized and controlled before anaesthesia and surgery to reduce the risks of rapidly varying swings in blood pressure. Surges of high blood pressure during procedures may cause angina, a heart attack or a stroke. Patients who have hypertension should be investigated for signs of damage to organs caused by the raised blood pressure. Organs often affected are the heart, brain and the kidneys.

Patients who have had a proven heart attack in the previous 6 months are usually considered unfit for non-urgent surgery, mainly because of the increased risk of another heart attack and death during or after the operation. Patients who have heart valve disease or who have had an artificial heart valve replacement have specific problems because they are often on drugs to prevent clots of blood forming on the valve or need antibiotics around the time of an operation. Patients with heart pacemakers require special care if surgical diathermy is to be used during the operation as electrical interference may cause the pacemaker to malfunction.

Respiratory system

One of the commonest reasons for patients being considered unfit for anaesthesia is because they have an acute respiratory infection. Anaesthesia may present risks to patients in that the infected secretions may get carried down into the lower airways and lungs. The vocal cords and lower airways are also very prone to spasm during anaesthesia if the patient has an active viral infection. This sensitivity of the respiratory tract lasts for 4–6 weeks. Acute viral illnesses may sensitize the heart muscle (myocardium) making it irritable and sometimes precipitating abnormal rhythms.

Asthma is associated with irritability and spasm of the airways. Patients with asthma are also more likely to suffer from allergies and more likely to develop sensitivity to drugs. Hypersensitivity of the airways means that secretions, suctioning, insertion of airways, laryngeal masks or endotracheal tubes can provoke spasm of the lower airways. Many of these patients are steroid dependent and may need steroid supplementation. During an asthma attack high airway pressures are needed to ventilate the lungs adequately and this results in a higher risk of development of a leak of air from the lung (pneumothorax).

The other common respiratory disease in the United Kingdom is chronic respiratory disease, which can be further classified as chronic *obstructive* airways disease (COAD) or chronic *restrictive* disease. In obstructive airways disease, the conducting airways are prone to spasm or narrowing. This presents as wheeze and bronchitis and is often associated with smoking. Restrictive lung disease affects the lung tissue, making it less elastic and less expandable. This can be associated with a number of diseases, including fibrosis. Patients with chronic lung disease are at greater risk than patients with healthy lung tissue because oxygen and carbon dioxide exchange is already impaired. Changes in the tissue of the lung and its blood supply during anaesthesia and surgery can further impair gas exchange. After surgery there may be other changes which may also worsen transfer of oxygen and carbon dioxide. It is important that the very best possible lung function is achieved before anaesthesia and surgery. These patients should stop smoking or, at the very least, not smoke on the day of surgery. Inhalation of nicotine paralyses the cells lining the respiratory tract and prevents the lung expelling the sticky secretions associated with smoking. This paralysis lasts from the first puff until about 30 minutes after the last puff. Effectively this means that a 20-a-day smoker has permanently paralysed lining cells during waking hours. Any chest infection must be treated with antibiotics and physiotherapy, and the physiotherapist can help to teach the patient deep-breathing exercises. Special techniques such as local anaesthetic blocks are often used to reduce the changes associated with anaesthesia and particular care is taken to relieve pain and to encourage adequate gas exchange and breathing after surgery. This is especially important after operations on the abdomen, chest or major bones.

PREMEDICATION

Premedicant drugs are given before an operation and have their effects before, during and after surgery. In the past, drugs were given to reduce some of the undesirable side effects of anaesthetic agents. For instance, an anaesthetic with ether caused lots of salivation and secretions. Changes in techniques and in the modern drugs now available mean very different premedications. The trend is now for premedication which relieves anxiety and is less sedative. This may worry some patients who may be fearful of being awake during the transfer to theatre. They may need considerable reassurance from ward and theatre staff that they will eventually be unconscious before surgery starts. The presence of a parent or guardian at induction of anaesthesia is helpful, especially in preschool children.

Some hospitals have a reception area for patients who can receive their premedicant drugs there and can await surgery under close supervision. More usually the premedication is given on the ward after all preparations for surgery have been completed. Remember that after the administration of premedicant drugs the patient is no longer held responsible for what they do. It is essential that the patient has given written consent for the operation before premedication is given. Clear instructions should be given not to leave bed following premedication. Some form of nurse call system must be in place in case assistance is needed for toileting or if the patient needs a nurse to speak to or feels unwell.

In addition to premedications, patients may need routine medication. Studies have shown that many essential drugs are omitted 'because the patient is fasting' yet oral premedicants are administered. Drugs which are particularly important include heart drugs (such as anti-arrythmics and beta blockers), drugs to help breathing (such as steroids or nebulizers) and drugs to control high blood pressure, angina, epilepsy or diabetes. Always check with the anaesthetist before omitting routine medications.

It is also very important that the premedication is properly prescribed, doubts checked with the prescribing doctor and the administration recorded in all the relevant documents. Theatre staff must check that the 'premed' has been given and, if not, check with the ward nurse and inform the anaesthetist.

Premedications are given

- to relieve anxiety;
- to treat or prevent pain;
- to reduce secretions;
- as part of the anaesthetic technique;
- to prevent postoperative sickness;
- to cause memory loss;
- to alter the stomach contents;
- to protect against reflexes which may slow the heart rate;
- to prevent the pain of injections.

Relief of Anxiety

The two main classes of drugs given for relief of anxiety are benzodiazepines and opioids. Benzodiazepines relieve anxiety and produce sleep, loss of memory and muscle relaxation. They may also reduce the likelihood of feeling sick or being sick (antiemetic effect). Given the night before surgery and on the day of surgery, they are safe, effective and useful. Usually they are given as tablets or capsules but they are also available in syrup form and can be given rectally as suppositories or by intramuscular or intravenous injection. Benzodiazepines used in anaesthetic practice include diazepam, temazepam, lorazepam and midazolam.

Pain Relief

Opioids produce pain relief, sleep and loss of memory. They are most effective in patients who already have pain. They do not specifically relieve anxiety but make the patient very sleepy. Usually opioids for premedication are given intramuscularly by injection, and often in conjunction with other drugs which reduce saliva and secretions or drugs to prevent sickness, to provide sleepy, comfortable pain-free patients. Examples of opioid drugs are morphine, diamorphine, papaveretum and pethidine. However, intramuscular injections are loathed by most children and their use should be avoided whenever possible. The non-steroidal anti-inflammatory drugs (e.g. diclofenac, ketorolac, ibuprofen, piroxicam, tenoxicam) can be given orally or by suppository as premedication to give analgesia and prevent the release of pain producing substances by tissues at the time of surgery.

Reduction in Secretions

Modern anaesthetic gases do not produce so much salivation and secretions and the use of drying agents or antisialogogues is much less common nowadays. For some types of surgery and during certain procedures there are advantages in having reduced saliva and secretions. Antisialogogues are used mainly in ear, nose and throat (ENT) surgery, oral and dental surgery and are frequently used if fibreoptic intubation is being performed. Hyoscine, atropine and glycopyrrolate are used. Hyoscine should be avoided in the elderly as it can cause confusion. Glycopyrrolate is more often used in patients with heart disease as it does not speed up the heart rate as much as atropine.

Part of the Anaesthetic Technique

Anaesthetists may order long acting drugs to be given before surgery so as to have their effect during or after the operation. Examples include beta blockers used to avoid fast heart rates in patients where it is planned to deliberately use a technique to lower the blood pressure, glyceryl trinitrate patches applied to prevent angina, and pain killers to give a degree of pain relief after surgery.

Memory Loss

In some patients memory loss is considered an advantage and drugs are given to achieve this. Examples include patients for cardiac surgery and some paediatric patients. Benzodiazepines provide amnesia and these are often given orally. An opioid given sometime later may be used to enhance this effect but care is required to prevent oversedation.

Modification of Stomach Contents

Patients at risk of regurgitation may receive drugs in an attempt to reduce the acidity and volume of stomach contents so that if aspiration into the lungs occurred, the damage to the lungs would be reduced. Pregnant patients, those with hiatus hernia and patients awaiting emergency surgery are particularly at risk. The gastric contents can be made less acid by giving antacids such as sodium citrate to neutralize the stomach acid and/or by giving histamine (H_2) receptor antagonists such as cimetidine or ranitidine which stop the secretion of acid from the stomach lining. Antacids (e.g. sodium citrate) neutralize the acid already in the stomach for 20–30 minutes. It is important that antacids should not contain solid particles as these can cause lung damage (e.g.

magnesium trisilicate). H_2 receptor antagonists prevent *further* acid from being produced but have no effect on the gastric contents at the time of administration. Metoclopromide and cisapride can also be used to encourage emptying of the stomach and so reduce the volume of the stomach secretions.

Correctly applied cricoid pressure must still be used, however, to stop spillover of gastric contents into the lungs (see pp. 60–5).

Protection Against Vagal Reflexes

Direct or indirect stimulation of the vagus nerve causes a slowing of the heart rate. The classic example is that of the eye surgeon pulling on an external eye muscle in a child having a squint correct which can cause a very slow heart rate or even cardiac arrest. Similar reflexes are now seen more commonly whenever traction is put on structures supplied by the vagus nerve lining the abdomen (the peritonium). The reason for this seems to be that modern anaesthetic drugs do not tend to speed up the heart rate and the effects of vagal stimulation are more readily seen. Atropine or glycopyrrolate are given to block this reflex response.

Prevention of Pain of Injections

Local anaesthetic creams are now available to anaesthetize the skin. EMLA cream is used commonly in children and is a mixture of two local anaesthetics namely lignocaine and prilocaine. It has to be applied 1 hour before the proposed injection in children and must be covered with a transparent film ('occlusive') dressing. This keeps the local anaesthetic in close contact with the skin and also tends to make the skin surface moist which improves the penetration of the local anaesthetic. Amethocaine gel ('Ametop') is a new form of an old local anaesthetic and is useful because it works quicker (30–45 minutes).

KEY LEARNING POINTS

1. Prepare the patient for anaesthesia and surgery as you would wish to be prepared yourself.
2. Individualize the preparation of each patient for age, maturity, level of understanding, communication ability, psychological state, medical condition, operation and type of anaesthesia.

3. Ensure all the preoperative checks are carried out and documented: if you are not satisfied, alert the anaesthetist and surgeon in charge of the case.

4. Premedication drugs are important but are only part of the overall preparation of the patient for anaesthesia and surgery.

Further Reading

1. Consent: 'Medical Ethics Today', British Medical Association. BMJ Publishing Group, London, 1993.
2. Fasting: Phillips S, Daborn AK, Hatch DJ 'Preoperative fasting for paediatric anaesthesia'. British Journal of Anaesthesia 1994; 73: 529–536.

Relevance

ODP Level 3 Units 0, 4, 5.

2. PREPARATION OF THE WORKPLACE AND EQUIPMENT

N. S. Morton, W. Davis

INTRODUCTION

'Be prepared' is an old-fashioned motto but in anaesthesia it is a very important principle. When things go wrong during anaesthesia the speed of change can be alarming and the need for intervention must often be immediate to avoid harm to the patient. A good example is a patient having an abdominal operation; on opening the peritoneum the heart rate can slow dramatically within a few seconds – the treatment must be immediate or the heart rate may slow to dangerously low levels. The surgeon should stop pulling on the peritoneum – this causes the stimulation of the vagus nerves which cause the heart rate to slow – and the anaesthetist should give an intravenous bolus dose of atropine which blocks the effects of the vagus nerve on the heart. Usually the heart rate immediately recovers and the surgery can proceed. But this rapid response is only possible with the modern standard of monitoring of the patient, with reliable access to the circulation and with atropine ready to give immediately. Thus preparation and checking of the equipment and drugs is, literally, vital for patient safety. It is ultimately the legal and professional responsibility of the anaesthetist in charge of the case to ensure that the anaesthetic and monitoring equipment is in working order, that appropriate drugs and fluids are available and given in the correct dose. However, the anaesthetist's assistant can help tremendously in a busy operating department and the anaesthetist will often work with the assistant in preparation of the workplace, drugs and equipment.

A good analogy is to think of an anaesthetic as an aircraft flight: the preparation phase is the 'pre-flight check' or 'cockpit drill', the induction of anaesthesia is the 'take-off', the maintenance of anaesthesia during the operation is the 'level flight' and the recovery from anaesthesia is the 'landing'.

THE ANAESTHETIC MACHINE

Today's anaesthetic machine/station (Figs 2.1 and 2.2) is based on a substantial, stable trolley. The trolley has to move relatively easily around the operating

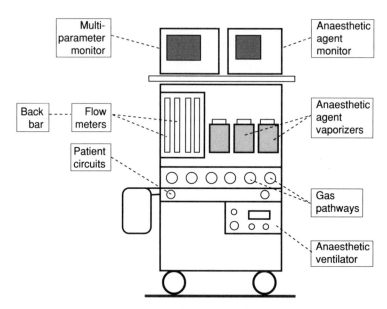

Fig. 2.1 Anaesthetic machine, front view

room and carry an average load of 200 kg. The primary design criteria, like a car, are performance, safety and operator comfort.

Pipeline Gas Supplies

Oxygen, nitrous oxide and medical air, along with vacuum and anaesthetic gas scavenging, are distributed by a network of degreased copper pipes throughout the hospital to wards and operating rooms, where they are terminated with colour-coded, self-closing, non-interchangeable supply outlet sockets (Fig. 2.2).

Pressures are measured in kilopascals (kPa). 100 kPa = 1 bar ≈ 1 atmosphere.

Oxygen, O_2

Liquid oxygen (at less than $-120°C$) is delivered once or twice a week by tanker to replenish the hospital storage tank. The 20 m^3 alloy steel vacuum flask/tank keeps the liquid oxygen cool. The liquid oxygen then passes through an evaporator, a coiled pipe at air temperature and a gas pressure regulator to supply the hospital with pressure-regulated (400 kPa) gaseous oxygen. Liquid oxygen storage is very efficient as it produces approximately 800 times its volume of gas, that is 20 m^3 produces 16 000 000 litres of gas.

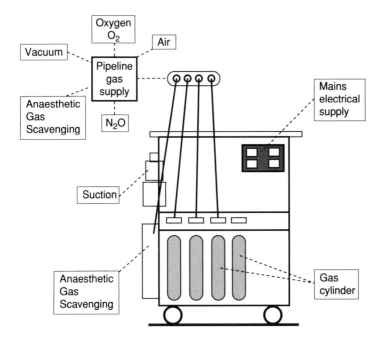

Fig. 2.2 *Anaesthetic machine, rear view*

There are also independent banks of large O_2 cylinders to backup the main liquid supply.

Air

Fresh air is filtered, compressed to 1000 kPa and stored in a large reservoir tank from where it is drawn off via dryers and further filtered, pressure regulated to either 700 kPa to drive surgical tools or 400 kPa for patient use. Most of the air plant is duplicated and there are normally two independent banks of large air cylinders to backup the plant.

Vacuum

The vacuum plant is virtually the air plant in reverse. A suction pump reduces the pressure in a large reservoir tank to 50 kPa below atmospheric pressure. This draws the exhaust from the hospital suction. Most of the vacuum plant is duplicated.

Anaesthetic Gas Scavenging (AGS)

The scavenging plant consists of a medium-sized suction pump or fan capable of drawing approximately 100 l/min from each anaesthetic site. The plant is duplicated to allow maintenance and backup. To protect staff and comply with 'Control of Substances Hazardous to Health' (COSHH) regulations it is mandatory to ensure that AGS is employed and operational. In the standard AGS system exhaled patient gases pass via a capped expiratory valve through a 30 mm diameter tube to an open-ended reservoir. The reservoir is continually emptied via a flow controller and indicator (normal flow 40 to 80 l/min) connected to the AGS pendant. It is essential that the AGS system does not obstruct or evacuate gas from the patient's breathing circuit.

Nitrous oxide, N_2O

Two banks of large cylinders containing a few days supply of liquid nitrous oxide are arranged so that one bank is 'in use' while the other is 'in reserve'. When the 'in use' bank empties, the reserve bank takes over. This is indicated (usually at the telephone exchange) then the empty cylinders are replaced and become the reserve bank. The N_2O manifold pressure is regulated to normal pipeline pressure (400 kPa).

Mains Electrical Supply

UK mains electricity is supplied at 50 Hz, 240 V. Should the mains fail, critical hospital areas are normally automatically (within 45 seconds) supplied by an emergency generator. A four socket, 2.5 A fused distribution box, connected to the mains via a 13 A fused socket supplies electricity to the anaesthetic machine. The above-mentioned fuses are intended to protect the equipment and cables and offer no patient or operator protection. Anaesthetic machine sockets are only intended for low current ventilators, monitors and infusion pumps. Suction pumps, heaters, diathermy, etc. will blow the fuses. Mains electricity supplied at 240 V and 13 or even 2.5 A can be extremely hazardous to patient and operator. 2.5 A equals 2500 mA. A 1 mA shock through your hand causes unpleasant tingling. A 25 mA shock throughout your body will cause pain, uncontrollable muscle contraction and possible ventricular fibrillation. Patients whose natural skin resistance is further reduced by ECG electrodes, needles and cannula, are further at risk from a fraction of 1 mA.

Suction

Where pipeline vacuum is available, the suction applied to the patient is controlled by a suction controller. The controller has an on/off switch, an adjustable knob and a gauge (high suction 0 to -100 kPa) to indicate the measured vacuum. To protect the controller and hospital vacuum from patient contamination a float stop valve and or a hydrophobic safety filter must be in circuit. High suction provides flows greater than 25 l/min and a vacuum greater than -70 kPa. A liquid collection container, with a float stop valve, must be situated between the patient and the controller.

Gas Cylinders

Gas cylinders are designed to safely store as much gas as possible in a small container. To achieve this the gas has to be forced into the cylinder under enormous pressure, for example O_2 and air at 13 500 kPa and N_2O and CO_2 at 5500 kPa (N_2O and CO_2 liquefy under pressure). Great care must be exercised when handling high-pressure cylinders containing anaesthetic gases. They must be opened carefully and as they may support combustion they must be free from oil, grease or any flammable substance. Cylinders are colour coded: O_2, black with white top; N_2O, blue; Entonox (50% N_2O/50% O_2 as liquid/gas premix), blue and white; CO_2, grey; air, grey with a black and white top; helium, brown. The anaesthetic machine cylinder holding yoke and respective cylinder are keyed (pin-indexed), allowing only the appropriate gas to enter. A high-pressure seal must be present between the cylinder and the yoke face and the cylinder must be opened two full turns. For liquids in cylinders (i.e. N_2O and CO_2) the pressure gauge does not start to fall until the cylinder is nearly empty (all the liquid has changed to gas).

Gas Pathways

Anaesthetic gases are available from two sources, primarily the hospital pipeline supply, backed up with machine-mounted high-pressure cylinders. Pipeline supplies, normally O_2, N_2O and air are delivered at 400 kPa, their presence being monitored by the pipeline gauges. High cylinder pressures are reduced and the pressure regulated to 400 kPa. Should the O_2 supply to the machine fail, the oxygen failure warning circuit will detect the reduced pressure and sound the alarm. Modern machines will also stop the delivery of N_2O, CO_2 and air to the patient. An O_2 bypass circuit ensures that, if a supply is available, emergency oxygen can be delivered directly to the common gas outlet. Some anaesthetic machines incorporate an on/off switch to connect the gas supplies to the flowmeters and the electrical supplies to the ventilator and/or monitors.

Flowmeters

The flow of gases between the supplies and the flowmeters are turned on and controlled by fine adjust needle valves. Each gas has an accurately calibrated ($\pm3\%$) variable orifice flowmeter. Improved low flow accuracy, for semi-closed circuit anaesthetics, can be obtained if two cascading flowmeters, a 0 to 1/min and a 1 to 10 l/min, are placed in series. Gas flow is read from the top of the rotating bobbin. The indicated flow will only be accurate if the flowmeter tube is vertical and the bobbin is rotating. Modern machines now incorporate a mandatory minimum safety O_2 to N_2O flow ratio, that is the patient gas always exceeds 25% O_2. The gas flow through the various flowmeter tubes mix in what is traditionally called the back bar.

Back Bar

The back bar is either a gas pipe which can readily be separated to accommodate anaesthetic agent vaporizers or a gas manifold with up to three sets of self-sealing inlet and outlet valve ports which allow easy selection of appropriately adapted vaporizers. Modern back bars and vaporizers incorporate a safety interlock mechanism to prevent simultaneous use of agents. As back bar pressure is 400 kPa great care must be exercised to ensure that all connections and seals are leak proof, as at 400 kPa all expected patient gas can be lost through a small leak. The prescribed vapour gas cocktail leaves the machine at the common gas outlet.

Anaesthetic Agent Vaporizers

Anaesthetic vaporizers (Fig. 2.3) add prescribed amounts of anaesthetic agent to the patient gas stream. All commonly used agents, halothane (red), enflurane (orange), isoflurane (purple), desflurane (blue) and sevoflurane (yellow), have clearly marked individually coloured vaporizers and all vaporizers are agent specific. A key filling system preventing agent spills and mix ups is strongly recommended. A large spill of liquid anaesthetic agent rapidly pollutes the air with dangerously high vapour levels; therefore, filling and draining should only be undertaken in a large, well-ventilated room. As agent metabolism has reduced with drug development, to minimize the risk from agent cross contamination it is recommended that the earlier developed agents are positioned at the right hand side, that is the downstream end, of the back bar.

Vaporizers range from reliable, temperature, flow and pressure compen-

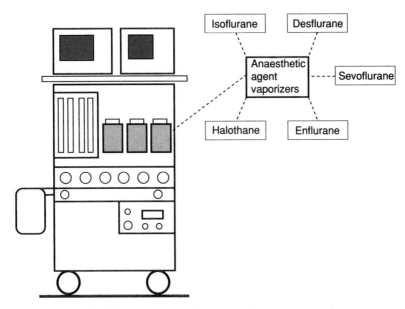

Fig. 2.3 *Anaesthetic machine, anaesthetic agent vaporizers*

sated mechanical units to electrically heated, electronically controlled, temperature, agent level, pressure monitored and alarmed units. Most vaporizers in use today are reliable and accurate over the normal anaesthesia maintenance range, 0.5% to 2% (desflurane 10%), 1 to 8 l/min, 18 to 28°C. They are less accurate at extremes. They are heavy (6 to 10 kg), dislike being tilted or dropped and should be stored in the area of use. Their liquid agent capacity ranges from 100 to 400 ml. All vaporizers should be drained from time to time to maintain agent purity. Halothane, in particular, if in constant use, should be drained into an appropriately marked container and discarded every few weeks when the agent level is low. New vaporizers tend to be heavier and some must not be used in the presence of flammable anaesthetics. As a 'rule of thumb' modern vaporizers should not be attached to old anaesthetic machines. Like our cars, vaporizers require to be serviced, some models once a year, some every three years. Occasionally vaporizers fail to give the expected output; fortunately this is usually detected by clinical observation. The increasing use of multi-gas/agent monitors will help this process.

Patient Circuits

The patient circuit is the tubing which delivers the prescribed anaesthetic gas/agent mixture produced in the anaesthetic machine to the patients lungs.

The four main circuits in common use are Magill, Bain, T-piece and circle (Figs 2.4 and 2.5). The restricted use of flammable anaesthetics allows the safe introduction of 'limited use' (one per list) plastic circuits and connectors with a 'disposable' (one per patient) filter heat and moisture exchanger (HME) at the patient connector. This reduces connection failure and improves the general hygiene of the procedure. It is now recommended that a new bacterial and viral filter is used for each patient to prevent cross infection.

An anaesthetic machine (nominal adult settings) produces a continuous 7 l/min flow of gas/agent mixture. During inspiration our lungs require a higher flow, 20 to 40 l/min and no flow during expiration. To match the gas supply to the patient's requirements a 2 l reservoir bag is incorporated into all commonly used adult patient circuits. During inspiration the reservoir bag empties, providing the short-term high flow required; during expiration the bag has time to refill. Circuits without reservoir bags require much higher gas flows.

Magill (Mapelson A) is a circuit consisting of a 2 l reservoir bag attached to the machine gas outlet, a single 1 meter length of corrugated tubing connected to a capped adjustable pressure limiting (APL) valve or spill/expiratory valve, terminated with a mask or endotracheal tube connector. (Fig 2.4) This popular, simple concept circuit works well with spontaneously breathing patients and with the aid of CO_2 monitoring can be finely tuned to minimize gas/agent waste. It is commonly used during induction and reversal of anaesthesia, the reservoir bag giving a reasonable indication of patient respiratory effort. It is not recommended for controlled ventilation as inspiratory gas is spilled via the APL valve. The coaxial version of the Magill circuit is the Lack circuit (Fig. 2.5).

Bain (Mapelson D) is a coaxial circuit in which the fresh anaesthetic gas/agent mixture flows through the inner tube to the patient connection end

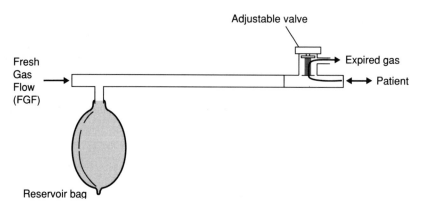

Fig. 2.4 Magill (Mapleson A) circuit: the most efficient for spontaneous breathing in adults

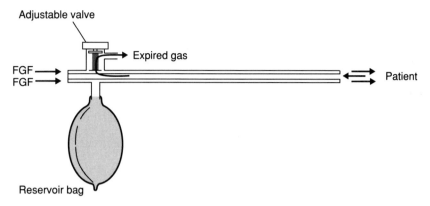

Fig. 2.5 Lack (Mapleson A) circuit: also very efficient in spontaneously breathing adults

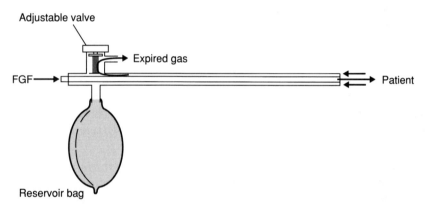

Fig. 2.6 Bain (Mapleson D): not so efficient for spontaneous breathing; good for controlled ventilation

and the exhaled patient gases pass back up the outer tube to the reservoir bag and capped APL valve at the machine end. (Fig 2.6) It is better for controlled ventilation than the Magill as its APL valve preferentially spills expired gases. It has the further advantage of the APL valve and associated scavenging tubing being away from the patient. It requires high gas/agent flows, up to twice the patients tidal volume in spontaneous mode, and as a coaxial circuit it requires frequent careful examination to insure that the inner tubing and connections are intact.

The Humphrey ADE circuit combines the benefits of the A for spontaneous breathing with the D for controlled ventilation. It has a lever to switch between the two systems and can be used in adults or children. It has an attachment point for scavenging anaesthetic gases.

Ayre's T-piece (Mapelson E/F) is normally only used with infants and is

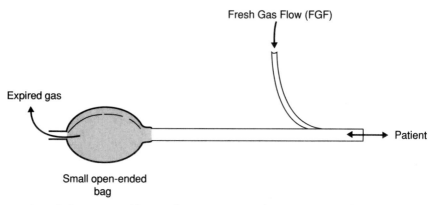

Fig. 2.7 F (Jackson–Rees modification of Ayres T-piece; – paediatric T-piece): best for children ≤20 kg

the simplest anaesthetic circuit as it has no APL valve. (Fig. 2.7) The fresh anaesthetic gas/agent mixture, similar to the Bain, is delivered directly at the patient connection end, therefore high flows, up to twice the tidal volume, are required to provide peak inspiratory flow demands and prevent rebreathing. Exhaled gases pass back out a large open-ended tube which may be terminated with a small open-ended reservoir bag to give an indication of respiratory effort. Intermittent manual closure of the bag exhaust allows controlled ventilation to be performed. Satisfactory scavenging is difficult.

Circle or closed circuit, is a patient gas/agent recycling (green) circuit. It is more an additional machine than a circuit, consisting of a reservoir bag, an APL valve and two intricate one-way valves to ensure gas circulation. A soda lime canister is also incorporated to remove exhaled CO_2 by absorption and a chemical reaction, which generates heat and water vapour. Recycling anaesthetic gases and expensive agents saves resources, causes less exhaust pollution and conserves patient gas heat and moisture. Once anaesthesia is established only small amounts of gas and agent require to be added to maintain anaesthesia. In practice, a safety margin of four times the minimum required level is usual. The large sodalime canister with its associated seals can be a source of circuit leaks. With the low gas flows involved the circuit should be pressure leak tested prior to each list. In-circuit gas and agent monitoring are strongly recommended with low fresh gas flow circle anaesthesia.

Anaesthetic Ventilators

A non-rebreathing automatic anaesthetic ventilator collects the gas/agent mixture produced in the anaesthetic machine into a bag/bellows, it then squeezes the bellows which forces the gas/agent mixture down one of two tubes connected to the patients lungs, while simultaneously blocking the other tube, expanding/ventilating the lungs. It then opens the blocked tube allowing the lungs to contract, whilst refilling its bellows.

The ventilator controls allow you to adjust:

- the amount of gas/agent mixture it collects in the bellows 'tidal volume' (TV)
- the speed with which the bellows is squeezed 'inspiratory flow'
- the number of times the bellows fill and empty in a minute 'rate/frequency' (Breaths/min)
- whether to fully or partially remove the blockage on the expiratory tubing 'positive end expiratory pressure' (PEEP).

A circle/rebreathing ventilator operates similarly but it primarily collects recycled gas/agents into its bellows.

Confusion is possible with multiple tubing connections (Spaghetti). Anaesthetic ventilators can have up to five connecting tubes requiring ten correct connections. Care must be exercised when making connections, particularly with units capable of ventilating both rebreathing and non-rebreathing circuits. Vigilance with APL valve setting is also required to avoid overpressuring the patient's lungs.

Monitoring and alarms

Various ventilator (machine) and patient parameter monitors with associated alarms are employed to inform and warn the operator of machine malfunction and any breach of patient alarm settings. Modern ventilators incorporate them, while older units require various separate add-on ventilator monitor alarms.

Typical machine warnings/alarms
- Mains power failure.
- Drive gas failure (whistle).
- Electronic self diagnostic failure.
- Control settings not achieved.
- Lack of gas/agent mixture, air entrainment.

Typical patient monitoring with alarm warnings
- Inspiratory oxygen concentration.
- Airway pressure. Low alarm which if not passed every 20 s will warn of ventilation failure or tubing disconnection.

- Upper alarm to warn, when incorporated within the ventilator, to stop excessive airway pressures occurring.
- Tidal volume, high and low.
- Minute volume, high and low.
- Breathing rate, inspiratory/expiratory (I:E) ratio.

Multi-parameter Patient Monitors

Monitors capable of measuring and recording the patient's ECG, oxygen saturation by pulse oximetry (SpO_2), invasive and non-invasive blood pressure (BP) and temperature are commonly either integrated into the anaesthetic machine or mounted on its top shelf, (Fig 2.7). The previous 5 to 10 s of measured parameters (ECG, SpO_2, BP) are displayed as waveforms on a screen. Measured and calculated values for heart rate, oxygen saturation, BP and temperature are displayed digitally and it is possible to set desired high and low alarm limits for each parameter. Clearly a machine capable of measuring five parameters and deriving over ten digital values with associated warning alarms is complex and requires appropriate operator training. Patients connected to mains electrically powered monitors, whose natural skin resistance is reduced by ECG electrodes, needles and cannula are at risk from a fraction of 1 mA of mains electrical current. Special patient electrical isolation is built into monitors to minimize the likelihood of patient electrocution, the integrity of which must periodically be tested. This isolation can be breached by an operator having an ungloved hand on the patient and the other on an electrically powered machine.

Electrocardiogram (ECG)

ECG is monitored to indicate the electrical activity of the patient's heart, that is rate, waveform, etc. It is a small electrical signal of about 1/1000th of a volt, produced by cardiac muscle contraction, measured at the patient's skin. Advanced amplifiers aid reliable measurement of this very small signal, even in the operating room environment with its high level of electrical interference. No amount of sophisticated electronics will overcome poor electrode application. A few seconds of skin preparation, examination of electrode gel and sensible electrode positioning are the basic essentials for obtaining a reliable ECG. Usual electrode positions are on the front of the upper right and left chest and over the apex of the heart.

Pulse oximeter (SpO_2)

SpO_2 measures the percentage of haemoglobin which is carrying oxygen.

This is achieved by shining red and infrared light through the finger or ear lobe. The absorption of light measured in vessels carrying pulsating arterial blood allows the computer in the pulse oximeter to calculate the SpO_2. Units are usually accurate to $\pm2\%$ over the 100% to 80% range. The pitch of the beep falls as the SpO_2 falls and rises as the SpO_2 rises. The measuring site should be checked every few hours on adults, and more frequently with children and patients with poor perfusion to minimize the risk of burns of the skin by the infrared probe.

Non-invasive blood pressure (NIBP)

An NIBP monitor is an automated cuff method of measuring patient's BP. The cuff is inflated above the predicted systolic pressure, then slowly deflated, and the systolic, diastolic and mean BP are derived from pressure measurements during cuff deflation. They can also be derived by an inflating cuff technique. They are accurate over the normal expected BP range and can be set to take a measurement at a variety of time intervals.

Invasive blood pressure (IBP)

IBP monitoring measures the actual pressure variations within the patient's circulatory system by directly connecting a pressure transducer via saline solution or inserting a miniature transducer on the tip of a catheter. The pressure transducer converts pressure variations into electrical signals, which are amplified and displayed as a waveform on the screen and from which systolic, diastolic and mean pressures are derived. Convenient, accurate, reliable, inexpensive, single-patient use pressure transducers which incorporate a fluid flushing device (Fig 2.8) and three-way tap are readily available.

IBP measurement procedure is as follows. A heparinized 500 ml bag of normal saline, pressurized to 300 mmHg by a bag pressure infuser, is connected and flushed through the transducer and tap, taking care to remove all air. The transducer is then interfaced to the patient via a saline-filled appropriate length of manometer line, three-way tap and canula. The transducer is then positioned as close as is practical to the level of the patient's heart.

Zeroing: with transducer tap closed to patient, transducer open to room air, initiate monitor zero.

Calibration: a quick calibration check may be performed by holding the patient end of the fluid-filled manometer line a measured height, for example 50 mmHg (68 cm or 27 inches), above the tap zero position.

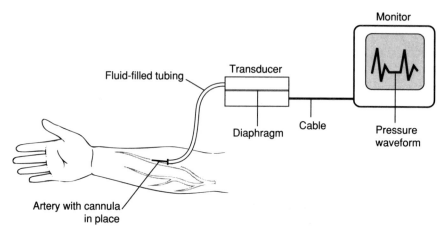

The pulse pressure wave travels along the fluid-filled tubing to the diaphragm, whose movement is converted (transduced) into an electrical signal which can be displayed on a monitor.

Fig. 2.8 Invasive blood pressure monitoring

Anaesthetic Gas/Agent Monitors

Anaesthetic machine, top shelf mounted or machine integrated, gas/agent monitors capable of measuring all commonly used gases and agents are readily available (Fig 2.9). They replace the stand alone CO_2, agent and O_2 monitors. They are accurate over clinical ranges, have selectable alarms, measure all required anaesthetic gas/agents, with calibration needed only every few months. They are side stream, that is gas is sampled as close as possible to the patients airway by drawing approximately 200 ml/min of gas through a sampling line into the analyser. Some heat and moisture exchange filters have useful sampling ports. The port is further from the airway than is preferred, especially for patients with a small tidal volume, but they have the protection of being upstream of the filter. The sample enters the analyser through a water trap. CO_2, N_2O and agents are measured by infrared absorption. Oxygen is measured either by a fuel-cell (slow, 20 s) or a paramagnetic sensor (fast, 0.5 s). As all other gases and agents are measured in 0.5 s, the faster paramagnetic O_2 measurements allows simultaneous continuous analyses of all gases/agents for patients breathing up to approximately 40 BPM. Calibration is performed by adjusting analyser readings to correspond with a sample from an accurate calibration gas canister. The analyser sample exhaust should either be connected to the scavenging system or, in low flow circle systems, be returned to the circuit.

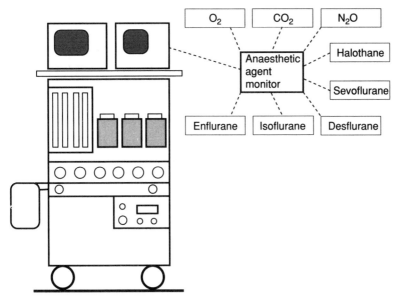

Fig. 2.9 Anaesthetic gas/agent monitors

Infusion Pumps

Three types of infusion pumps are used by anaesthetists.

- Syringe drivers, which utilize an electronically controlled electric motor to drive the plastic syringe plunger, infusing the syringe contents into the patient.
- Volumetric, which utilize a peristaltic action or piston cassette pump insert to control the prescribed infusion volume.
- Patient controlled analgesia (PCA) device, which is a syringe driver that allows the patient, within defined limits, to control their own drug delivery (see pp. 187–93).

Syringe drivers replace the doctor/nurse's thumb by controlling the speed and the distance (flow rate and volume infused) that the syringe plunger is pushed. The operator must use the correct size of syringe, make sure it is properly in place and frequently monitor that it is delivering the expected drug dosage. Syringe drivers administer up to 100 ml of drug at flow rates of 0.1 to 100 ml/h.

Volumetric infusion pumps are used to administer intravascular drugs, fluids, whole blood and blood products accurately. They can administer up to 2000 ml of fluid (normally from a bag or bottle) at flow rates of 0.1 to 2000 ml/h.

PCA pumps utilize a patient hand control, which when pressed, delivers a pre-set bolus of analgesic drug. Immediately after delivery the pump will refuse to deliver another bolus until a pre-set time has passed. The pre-set bolus size and lockout time, along with background (constant drug infusion) are pre-programmed by the doctor.

Many pumps operate from battery and mains electricity. They incorporate warnings and alarms of excessive upstream pressure, air in tube, syringe empty/nearly empty and low battery. Normally the total volume of fluid to be delivered can be set, and following delivery, an end of infusion, KVO (keep vein open) flow of 1 to 2 ml/h will continue to infuse.

Modern infusion pumps (clever as they are) require frequent monitoring to ensure that they are delivering the prescribed treatment. Free flow of fluid due to incorrect housing of pump insert or syringe is a common cause of severe over-infusion.

Blood/Fluid Warmer

Traditionally, infused blood and fluids were warmed by passing them through a plastic coil heat exchanger in a temperature-controlled water bath. There was a risk of spillage of hot water and electric shock from these devices and they are not very efficient at high infusion rates. To remove the problems associated with water baths, dry warmers were introduced, where the plastic coil (sometimes flattened) is heated by metal heat exchangers (temperature controlled metal plates).

Rapid fluid warming can be achieved by using highly efficient, jacketed heat exchangers, where the patient's fluid passes through the inner tube and water heated to a maximum of 37°C in a tank is pumped through the outer jacket.

Dry warmers can raise cold fluid temperatures to 35°C at a flow of 75 ml/min. Rapid warmers can raise cold fluid temperatures to 35°C at a flow of 500 ml/min. Modern fluid warmers are set to operate at 37°C; if their temperature rise above 40°C heating stops and an alarm is sounded.

Diathermy

Diathermy is of anaesthetic interest as it can interfere with vital monitoring, pacemaker operation and cause unintentional patient burns.

Normal (monopolar) diathermy depends on passing a high voltage (3000 to 8000 V) high-frequency (1 MHz) current into the patient's body via a *small* tipped instrument, with the current passing through the body tissues and returning to the diathermy via a *large* body surface area contact plate. The same current flows through both patient connections, and the local cutting and coagulation effect at the active connection is due to the higher current density i.e. the energy is concentrated into a small area. If the large return plate connection is poorly applied then its contact with the patient may reduce in area causing patient burns under the plate. Modern diathermys have plate contact monitoring and patient earthing alarms which should not be ignored.

Diathermy interference on monitoring and pacemaker operation may be reduced by ensuring that patient connections are distanced from the diathermy patient current path. The interference risks to monitoring and pacemaker operation are much reduced with bipolar diathermy where the current passes from one blade of a pair of forceps to the other. No current passes through the patient's body with this technique except for the piece of tissue grasped by the forceps. It is only suitable for local coagulation of small areas.

Argon diathermy is a unipolar diathermy with the addition of a stream of argon gas. This ionizes and produces a stream of energized particles which can cut and coagulate tissues. This has the advantage of using lower power and yet producing a more focused area of tissue damage.

Defibrillator

Defibrillators are used to treat patients in ventricular fibrillation, to cardiovert (restore normal heart rhythm) and to restart the heart following cardiopulmonary bypass surgery.

Adult ventricular fibrillation is treated by:

1 Initially setting the defribillators delivered output charge to approximately 250 joules.
2 Applying electrode contact paste/gel to both paddles, or utilizing defibrillator contact pads (pads reduce the risk of the charge passing over the skin due to an excess of contact gel).
3 Placing the paddles firmly onto the patients front chest wall, (sternum) to the patients upper right chest and (apex) to the patients lower left chest.
4 Charging the defibrillator to the previously set output charge.
5 Pressing the firing switch (normally two buttons, one on each paddle) then passes the stored, approximately 3000 V 30 A charge through the patient's heart.
6 Should the initial recommended average adult setting not be effective, the output setting is increased.

WARNING   defibrillators deliver a 5000 V 50 A electric shock. Beware nitrate patches (ETN) which are used to treat angina as these could explode if this current is applied to them.

It is *essential* that good electrical contact is obtained, but *only* immediately under the paddle/pad and that the operator and any other staff are well insulated (distanced and not touching) from the defibrillator, patient and bed/table.

Cardioversion is achieved by synchronizing the defibrillator firing with the patient's ECG R wave.

Child external, and adult internal defibrillation may be limited to a maximum output setting of 100 joules. The normal child external setting is 2 to 4 joules/kg.

AN ALPHABETICAL CHECKLIST FOR ANAESTHESIA EQUIPMENT

A   Airway

Suction apparatus; laryngoscopes; intubation aids; endotracheal tubes; airways laryngeal masks; masks.

B   Breathing

Breathing circuits; ventilators; vaporizers; anaesthetic machine; humidifiers; heat and moisture exchangers.

C   Circulation

Venous cannulation; central venous cannulation, arterial cannulation, transducers; blood and fluid warmers; pulmonary artery catheters; pacemaker equipment.

D   Drugs

General anaesthesia; local anaesthesia; antiemetics; circulatory support; muscle relaxants; analgesics; resuscitation; respiratory support; specialized drugs; antibiotics; drugs to treat anaphylaxis.

CHECKING THE ANAESTHETIC MACHINE

This pictoral check is derived and extended from *Checklist for Anaesthetic Machines: a recomended procedure based on the use of an oxygen analyzer* published July 1990 by the Association of Anaesthetists of Great Britain & Ireland, 9 Bedford Square, London WC1B 3RA. The original document must have been read previously. Easy modifications may be made if there is no pipeline supply or a varying number of cylinders.

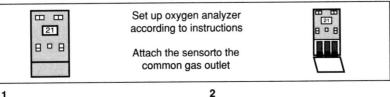

Set up oxygen analyzer according to instructions

Attach the sensor to the common gas outlet

1   2

Medical Gas Supplies

- Anaesthetic machine disconnected from pipelines
- Remove all unwanted cylinders
- Check remaining cylinders correctly seated and turned "off"
- Empty yokes blanked
- All vaporizers "off"
- Electrical supply "on"
- Open ALL flowmeter control valves

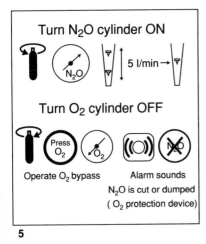

Turn O₂ cylinder ON

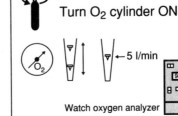

←5 l/min

Watch oxygen analyzer

3   4

Turn N₂O cylinder ON

5 l/min→

Turn O₂ cylinder OFF

Press O₂

Operate O₂ bypass   Alarm sounds
                         N₂O is cut or dumped
                         (O₂ protection device)

Connect the oxygen pipeline

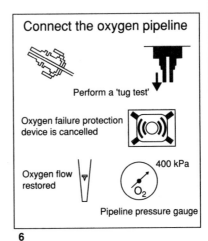

Perform a 'tug test'

Oxygen failure protection device is cancelled

Oxygen flow restored

400 kPa

Pipeline pressure gauge

5   6

Fig. 2.10 Checking the anaesthetic machine (reproduced with permission of Professor AP Adams)

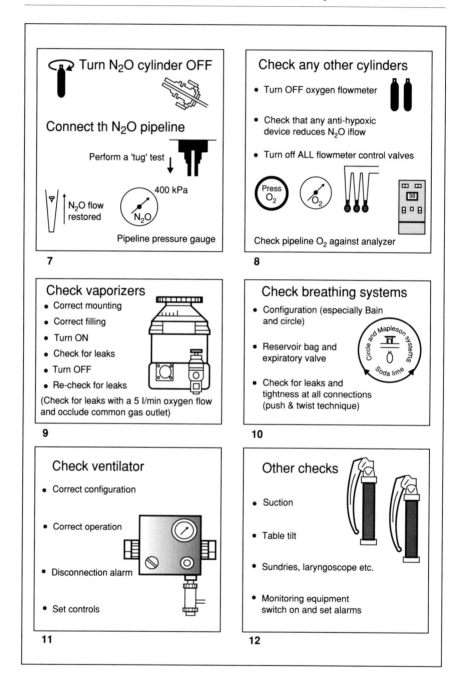

Fig. 2.10 Checking the anaesthetic machine (cont.)

E1 Electrical

Monitoring; defibrillator; electrosurgical; nerve stimulator; diathermy.

E2 Environment

Tables and attachments; trolleys, warming mattress, infection control; patient eye protection; padding and pressure area care.

F Fluids

Fluids; infusion pumps; blood and blood products; fluid warming equipment.

This checklist can help you to ensure you have attended to all the important items. A useful check for correct functioning of the anaesthetic machine is that recommended by the Association of Anaesthetists (Fig 2.10).

KEY LEARNING POINTS

1. Be prepared by using a cockpit drill and checklist.
2. Know where things are in your workplace or how to get them quickly.
3. Discuss each case with the anaesthetist in advance so you can anticipate routine requirements, unusual requirements and emergency needs.
4. Alert the anaesthetist if equipment appears faulty or is unavailable.
5. The ultimate legal responsibility for equipment, drugs and fluids rests with the anaesthetist.

Further Reading

'Ward's Anaesthetic Equipment', 3rd edition. Davey A, Moyle JTB, Ward CS. WB Saunders, London, 1992.
'Essentials of Anaesthetic Equipment', Baha Al-S, Simon S. Churchill Livingstone, London, 1995.

Relevance

ODP Level 3   Units 0, 1, 2, 3.

SECTION 2
INDUCTION OF ANAESTHESIA

3. INDUCTION OF GENERAL ANAESTHESIA

C. J. Runcie, G. Gillies

THE STRAIGHTFORWARD INDUCTION IN AN ELECTIVE CASE

Until the 1840s, operations were performed without any anaesthetic. In that decade, the anaesthetic gas nitrous oxide and the anaesthetic vapour ether were demonstrated for the first time. Intravenous anaesthetic drugs were first used in the 1930s and muscle relaxant drugs in the 1940s. Modern concepts of anaesthesia date from that time.

General anaesthesia can be divided into three components – unconsciousness (hypnosis), pain relief (analgesia) and muscle relaxation. Specific drugs are given for specific components. Thus intravenous anaesthetics and anaesthetic gases ensure hypnosis, opiate drugs relieve pain and muscle relaxant drugs provide muscular paralysis, allowing the surgeon access to body cavities like the abdomen. Doses of each drug can therefore be kept to a safe minimum.

In the early days these three objectives were achieved using only one drug, an anaesthetic gas or vapour. To achieve adequate muscle relaxation, large amounts of anaesthetic gas had to be given which was risky for all but the fittest of patients.

The Stages of Anaesthesia

All anaesthetic drugs produce anaesthesia by their effect on the brain. Anaesthetic gases are inhaled and then must be transferred from the lungs to the circulation and finally to the brain to be effective. Administering an anaesthetic gas *alone*, the progress of the patient towards deep anaesthesia is divided into four stages.

- *Stage 1* is the stage of *analgesia* and lasts from the beginning of administration of the gas until consciousness is lost.
- *Stage 2* is the stage of *excitement*, lasting from loss of consciousness until

settled regular breathing begins. During this period the patient may struggle, breath hold, vomit or cough.

- *Stage 3.* Once settled regular breathing has begun, the stage of *surgical anaesthesia* has been reached and the operation may begin.
- *Stage 4.* If more anaesthetic is given, the patient enters the fourth stage (of *overdosage*) and his breathing and circulation will ultimately stop.

This sequence of events was common when only anaesthetic gases were available. Induction of anaesthesia was prolonged and its stages clear cut. Intravenous anaesthetic drugs are now used to induce anaesthesia. They are carried quickly to the brain and surgical anaesthesia is reached more rapidly and the other stages of anaesthesia are less obvious. It is still helpful to know about the stages of anaesthesia because induction by anaesthetic gas (an inhalational induction) remains the preferred technique for some patients and situations. Understanding the problems of the second stage of excitement allows them to be anticipated and dealt with more easily.

Drugs for inhalational induction of anaesthesia

Halothane is the most commonly used volatile anaesthetic agent for inhalational induction in children or in patients with difficult or irritable airways. This is because it is a hydrocarbon molecule not an ether. It is relatively pleasant smelling and is non-irritant to the airway. The other volatile agents enflurane, isoflurane and desflurane are all ethers and have unpleasant smells and are irritant.

Sevoflurane is the least pungent and irritant of the volatile ethers and rivals halothane for inhalational induction in children. It has yet to be evaluated in the patient with the difficult airway.

Oxygen is of course used to carry these volatile agents and 100% oxygen is recommended in the difficult airway case. In patients with airway obstruction helium can be added to the oxygen/volatile agent mixture as its low density makes it easier to breath. In the child with a normal airway, nitrous oxide is often introduced along with oxygen to disguise the smell of the volatile agent and to speed up the induction.

INTRAVENOUS INDUCTION OF ANAESTHESIA

Conduct of Intravenous Induction

Adequate preparation is essential before intravenous (i.v.) induction of anaesthesia. Chapters 1 and 2 describe the preparation of anaesthetic equipment. This must include equipment for urgent tracheal intubation plus the relevant drugs, that is suxamethonium and atropine. Other drugs are drawn up by the anaesthetist as appropriate.

Once the patient has arrived in the anaesthetic or operating room and the routine preoperative checks have been completed, non-invasive monitors are applied. These are usually a pulse oximeter, electrocardiogram and non-invasive BP monitor. For specialized surgery, other monitors may be required.

Anaesthesia of the skin with local anaesthetic cream is particularly important in children or in very anxious adults (see Chapter 30). i.v. access is usually established by inserting a cannula into a vein in the forearm or back of the hand. A tourniquet is applied to the arm, a vein selected and antiseptic skin preparation applied, usually with a small single-use alcohol impregnated swab (e.g. Mediswab). Subcutaneous infiltration of the local anaesthetic lignocaine, 1 or 2% plain solution may be carried out using a fine 25 or 27G needle. Stinging can be minimized by using warmed local anaesthetic and by very slow injection. Once the cannula is secure and readings obtained from the monitors, the patient is preoxygenated. The patient breathes 100% oxygen for 3 minutes via a breathing system and face mask. 100% oxygen can only be administered if there is a good seal between the patient's face and the mask; the reservoir bag must be full.

A small test dose of the induction agent is then injected and its effects observed. Further drug is given according to the patient's response until surgical anaesthesia is achieved. The delay between injection and response is the time taken for the drug to be carried in the circulation from the arm to the brain – about 30 seconds in fit patients but much longer in old patients or those with a slow circulation due to poor heart function or low circulating volume (e.g. due to blood loss or dehydration).

Following i.v. induction, anaesthesia is maintained with inhaled anaesthetic gases and volatile agents. A mixture of nitrous oxide and oxygen is supplemented with a volatile agent – halothane, enflurane, isoflurane, desflurane or sevoflurane. Commonly, a laryngeal mask airway (LMA) is inserted after i.v. induction and the patient breathes anaesthetic gases via the LMA. A facemask and oral airway can be used for short cases. If muscle relaxant drugs are given, a tracheal tube can be passed and the patient's lungs mechanically ventilated with anaesthetic gases and oxygen.

The steps involved in i.v. induction are summarised in Figure 3.1.

The Intravenous Anaesthetic Drugs

Propofol (diisopropylphenol) is the most popular i.v. induction agent. In a

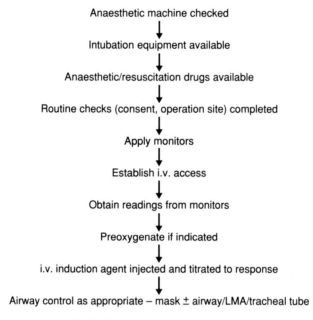

Fig. 3.1 *Sequence of events during i.v. induction*

dose of 2–2.5 mg/kg it acts rapidly, in one arm–brain circulation time. Its action is terminated by transfer from the brain to the tissues and metabolism by liver and plasma esterases. Patients regain consciousness about 5 minutes after drug injection.

Advantages

Propofol depresses airway reflexes so that an oral airway or LMA may be inserted immediately after induction. If this is attempted with the other induction agents, coughing and laryngospasm may ensue. Similarly, volatile agents can be promptly introduced at high concentration after propofol induction, allowing a rapid increase in lung and brain concentrations.

Propofol's other main advantage is rapid clear emergence from anaesthesia without any hangover effect, making it useful for day case procedures. It does not accumulate in the blood if given by continuous infusion and infusions are increasingly used to maintain anaesthesia while avoiding the side-effects of the volatile agents. It also has antiemetic effects and does not cause anaphylactic reactions.

Disadvantages

Hypotension following propofol is more marked than with other drugs. It is mainly due to vasodilation and particularly affects the elderly. Propofol is also a potent respiratory depressant; apnoea frequently follows induction. Minor problems include excitatory phenomena (twitching movements) and pain on injection. The latter is reduced by adding lignocaine, 0.1–0.2 mg/kg, to the syringe or by warming the propofol solution to body temperature immediately prior to injection. Preinjection of alfentanil, a short acting opioid, also helps injection pain. Bacteria can grow in propofol so open ampoules should be discarded and the solution should be given to the patient immediately after being drawn up.

Sodium thiopentone is a barbiturate induction agent in use since the 1930s. It comes in a powder form and is constituted with water for injection to a concentration of 25 mg/ml (2.5%). The induction dose is usually 1–5 mg/kg. It causes dose-related cardiovascular and respiratory depression and recovery may be quite prolonged.

Etomidate is useful in cardiac surgery or in patients with cardiovascular disease as it depresses the heart and circulation less than other drugs. It is also useful in the patient with severe asthma. Pain on injection is also a problem with this drug and the measures noted above for propofol are effective. It can produce involuntary movements and when given by infusion it switches off hormone production from the adrenal gland.

Airway Maintenance

Under anaesthesia, patients lose muscular tone, i.e., their limbs and abdominal muscles become lax and floppy. The muscles of the throat are similarly affected. Normally, the tone of these muscles holds the soft palate, tongue and epiglottis away from the back wall of the throat. Air can pass freely from the lungs to the mouth and vice versa. Induction of anaesthesia causes the soft palate, tongue and epiglottis to move toward the back wall of

Table 3.1

CLINICAL SIGNS OF AIRWAY OBSTRUCTION
Noisy breathing (snoring)
Indrawing of suprasternal notch and above clavicle
See-sawing of the abdomen and chest (as respiratory muscle effort increased to overcome the obstruction) (see Fig. 5.1)
Tracheal tug (pulling down of the larynx and trachea with each inspiration)
Reduced movement of the reservoir bag
Increasing cyanosis (blueness)

the throat. During inspiration the walls of the throat then collapse and the patient's airway becomes obstructed (Fig. 3.2).

Recognition and treatment of airway obstruction must be rapid and its signs are listed in Table 3.1. There are a variety of simple techniques to clear the airway. Turning the patient on his side is valuable regardless of the technique used.

Chin lift/jaw thrust

This involves extending the head on the neck by lifting the chin up (Fig. 3.3). This draws the tissues at the front of the neck taut and pulls them off the back wall of the throat.

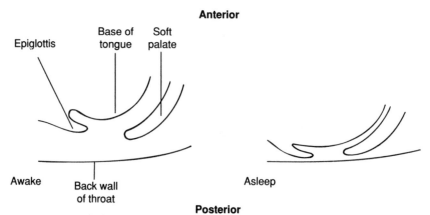

Fig. 3.2 Collapse of the airway under anaesthesia. The soft palate, base of tongue, epiglottis and posterior pharyngeal wall are shown (a) before and (b) after induction of anaesthesia

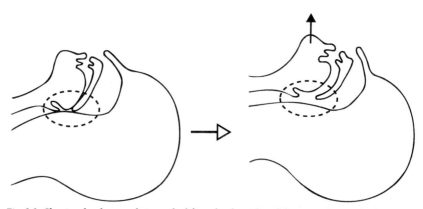

Fig. 3.3 Clearing the obstructed airway by lifting the chin. The solid arrow indicates the direction in which force is applied. The highlighted area is illustrated in more detail in Fig. 3.2

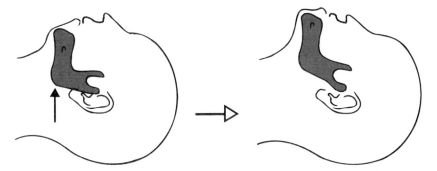

Fig. 3.4 The jaw thrust – clearing the airway by lifting the mandible in the direction of the arrow

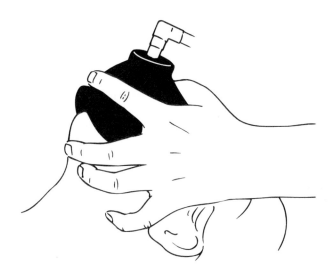

Fig. 3.5 Holding the anaesthetic face-mask in position

The next step is lifting the jaw directly upwards (jaw thrust), which is a two-handed manoeuvre (Fig. 3.4). Put your index and middle fingers behind the angles of the jaw and lift the jaw straight up towards the ceiling so that the lower jaw projects beyond the upper jaw. As with the chin lift, this lifts the structures at the front of the neck away from the back wall of the throat.

During an anaesthetic, the airway must be held open while anaesthetic gas is delivered via a breathing system and facemask (Fig. 3.5). The thumb and index finger press the facemask down while the middle and ring fingers pull the chin up. The little finger hooks round the angle of the jaw to lift the jaw directly upwards if necessary. The other hand can lift the angle of the jaw on the other side directly upwards also.

Oral airway

The Guedel oral airway (Fig. 3.6) acts by holding the tongue away from the back wall of the throat and separating the soft palate from the tongue. In adults it is inserted upside-down and rotated into its normal position as it passes backwards in the mouth. In children, it is inserted correct way up as there as there is less space to rotate the airway in the mouth.

Nasopharyngeal airway

This is passed through a nostril and holds the soft palate and tongue away from the back wall of the throat (Fig. 3.7). It must be lubricated well and inserted gently to avoid a nose bleed and is more easily tolerated by lightly anaesthetized patients than an oral airway. It should not be used in patients with a basal skull fracture or fracture of the middle one third of the face.

Laryngeal mask airway (LMA)

A conventional facemask forms a seal around the mouth and nose. In contrast, a laryngeal mask airway forms a seal around the opening of the larynx. The stem portion of the LMA passes up through the throat and emerges from the mouth. A breathing system is attached and anaesthetic gases inhaled through it. The correct size is shown in Table 3.2.

During insertion of the LMA, the tip of the mask must be pressed flat against the palate. As the LMA is inserted, one hand holds the head in good

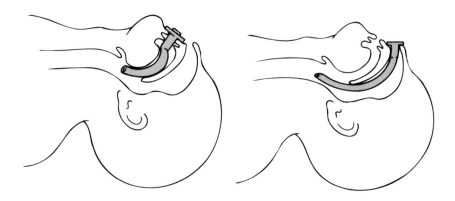

Fig. 3.6 A Guedel oral airway in position   *Fig. 37 A nasopharyngeal airway in position*

Table 3.2

LMA SIZES		
WEIGHT	**SIZE**	**CUFF INFLATION VOLUME**
up to 6.5 kg	1	2–4 ml
6.5–15 kg	2	10 ml
15–30 kg	2.5	15 ml
30–50 kg	3	20 ml
50–75 kg	4	30 ml
>75 kg	5	40 ml

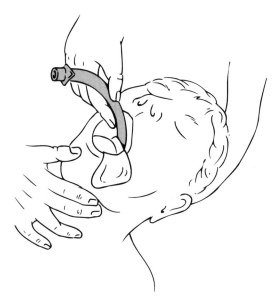

Fig. 3.8 Laryngeal mask airway

position and the other passes the LMA. An assistant should thus pull the lower jaw sufficiently far down to allow the LMA to pass into the mouth and prevent the lower lip being drawn over the teeth (Fig. 3.8). Finally, the LMA cuff should be inflated after insertion and *before* a breathing system is attached as this centres the LMA in good position in the throat (Fig. 3.9).

The flexible, reinforced LMA has a tube with a spiral wire in its wall to stop it kinking and is useful for head and neck, ENT, and eye cases.

The cuff of the LMA does not form a watertight seal around the laryngeal opening. Gastric contents can thus pass up the oesophagus, past the cuff of the LMA and down into the lungs. Only a tracheal tube can give the water-

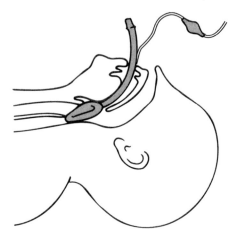

Fig. 3.9 A laryngeal mask airway forming a seal round the opening of the larynx. Compare this with the seal an anaesthetic face-mask forms around the mouth and nose in Fig. 3.5

tight seal necessary to prevent this. Laryngeal masks are therefore not suitable when there is a risk of regurgitation.

Tracheal Intubation

Tracheal intubation is the insertion of a breathing tube into the trachea through the vocal cords. This is normally performed under direct vision with the aid of a laryngoscope. The tube is usually passed through the mouth (oro-tracheal intubation), occasionally it is passed through the nose (naso-tracheal intubation) to allow surgical access to the mouth. The laryngoscope blade most commonly used is the curved Macintosh (Fig. 3.10) but a straight blade is often used in small children or in difficult intubations. The McCoy blade has a flexible tip which can help when intubation is difficult.

Most tracheal tubes used for adults have a gentle curve to ease placement and have an inflatable cuff at the distal end to provide an air-tight fit within the trachea (Fig. 3.11). Tracheal tube sizes refer to the internal diameter of the tube in millimetres.

A tube in the size range 7–9 would normally be used for oro-tracheal intubation in adults. Generally men require a larger tube than women. A suitable length for oro-tracheal tubes for adults would be 21–24 cm. (Table 3.3) Some operative procedures require the use of a special tube. These are described in the specialist chapters.

There are a number of specific indications for tracheal intubation for general anaesthesia.

Table 3.3

ENDOTRACHEAL TUBE SIZES			
AGE	WEIGHT (kg)	INTERNAL DIAMETER (mm)	UNCUFFED/CUFFED
Newborn	1–3	3.0	uncuffed
1 y	10	4.0	uncuffed
5 y	18	5.0	uncuffed
10 y	30	6.5	uncuffed/cuffed
15 y	50	7.5	cuffed
Adult	60	9.0	cuffed
Adult	70	9.0	cuffed

These sizes are a guide only.

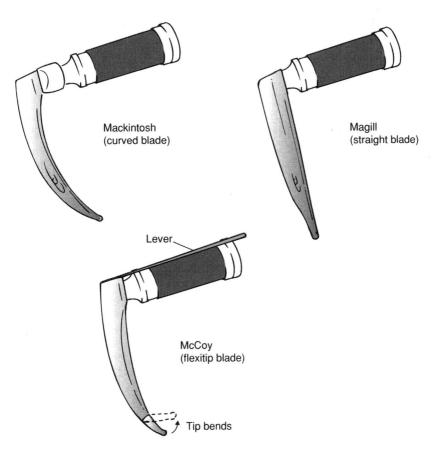

Mackintosh
(curved blade)

Magill
(straight blade)

Lever

McCoy
(flexitip blade)

Tip bends

Fig. 3.10 Types of laryngoscopes

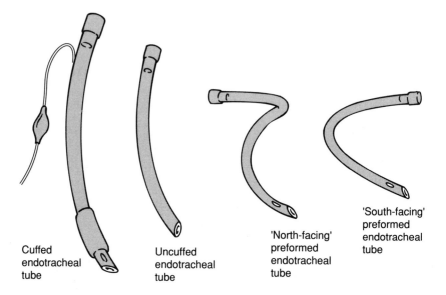

Cuffed
endotracheal
tube

Uncuffed
endotracheal
tube

'North-facing'
preformed
endotracheal
tube

'South-facing'
preformed
endotracheal
tube

Fig. 3.11 Endotracheal tube

1. To protect the airway
   - This is important for patients at risk of aspirating gastric contents, see Table 3.4.
   - Intubation is also indicated for surgery to the nose or mouth to protect the lungs from soiling with blood, pus or debris from above.
2. To allow surgical access. A tracheal tube provides a secure airway where anaesthetic access is limited, for example surgery to the head or neck.
3. To facilitate mechanical ventilation of the lungs
   - where muscle relaxation is required, for example for abdominal surgery;
   - where the work of breathing would be high, for example obesity, head down tilt or prone (face down) position;
   - to prevent the normal rise of CO_2 associated with spontaneously breathing general anaesthesia, for example in neurosurgery.

Equipment

To perform tracheal intubation safely, the following items of equipment are essential. It is important that all times of equipment are tested before use.
1. Source of suction with appropriate hand piece
2. Facemask and guedel airway of appropriate size
3. Tracheal tube of appropriate size and length prepared
4. Tracheal tube of smaller size available
5. Two laryngoscopes with a range of blade sizes and shapes

6. Syringe for inflation of tracheal cuff
7. Tracheal tube connector
8. Apparatus for applying positive pressure ventilation
9. Maleable introducer for altering endotracheal tube shape and gum elastic bougies for use as a guide.

In addition to the above it is good practice to have reasonable access to a difficult intubation kit and a flexible fibreoptic intubating laryngoscope, which may prove useful for an unpredicted difficult intubation (see p. 61–5).

Method of Laryngoscopy for Tracheal Intubation

Laryngoscopy for tracheal intubation is most easily performed with the patient in the correct position. In the neutral position the axis of the larynx, the pharynx, and the mouth are at quite different angles. (Fig. 3.12) Putting a head support or thick pillow behind the patient's head in the supine position flexes the neck and brings the axis of the larynx and pharynx into alignment (Fig. 3.13).

If the head is then extended at the atlanto-occipital joint, the axis of the mouth is brought into alignment with the axis of the larynx and pharynx and the patient is in the ideal position for laryngoscopy (Fig. 3.14).

For intubation with the Macintosh laryngoscope, the scope is held in the left hand and the blade is introduced into the right-hand side of the patient's mouth. The blade is then advanced into the oropharynx and swept towards the midline as it is advanced down the pharynx. In so doing, the flange on the left-hand side of the blade holds the distal part of the tongue to the left side of

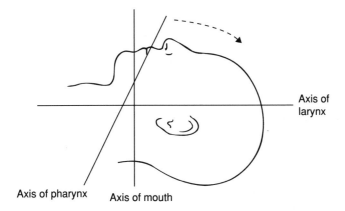

Fig. 3.12 *Axes are different so viewing larynx is very difficult*

the mouth. As the laryngoscope is advanced over the back of the tongue, the epiglottis comes into view.

The tip of the blade is then advanced into the vallecula which is the recess between the epiglottis and the base of the tongue. Once the tip of the scope is in the vallecula, the tongue and epiglottis are lifted by applying a moderate force in the direction of the handle. This reveals the larynx with its two vocal cords which have a white appearance. It is important that the laryngoscopy handle is not levered backwards as this might apply force to the upper teeth and would not improve the view. If the patient is paralysed the vocal cords are in a position of abduction (open) and form the shape of the letter 'A'.

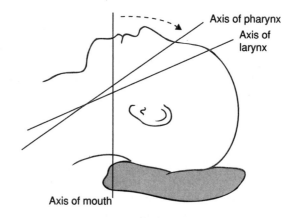

Fig. 3.13 Pillow brings 2 out of 3 axes into line

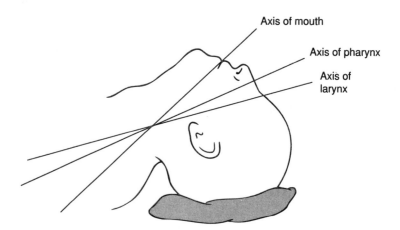

Fig. 3.14 All 3 axes are nearly in line so viewing larynx is much easier

Once a good view of the larynx is obtained, a tracheal tube can be advanced down the right side of the blade, through the larynx and into the trachea. The cuff is then inflated until there is a modest pressure palpable at the pilot balloon and no leak around the tube can be heard on applying positive pressure ventilation. Once the cuff is inflated, the anaesthetist listens to the chest with a stethoscope (auscultation) whilst applying a few breaths of positive pressure ventilation to check that the breath sounds are audible, equal on each side and louder over the lateral aspects of the chest than over the stomach. This ensures that the tip of the endotracheal tube is in the trachea and has not been advanced into one or other main bronchus or inadvertently placed behind the larynx into the oesophagus.

Auscultation is not an infallible test for detecting misplacement of the endotracheal tube. A flat end-tidal CO_2 monitor tracing is a more reliable method of detecting oesophageal intubation. A fibre optic bronchoscope can also be used to quickly check tube position if available.

Proficient assistance during laryngoscopy and tracheal intubation requires concentration and anticipation. All equipment should be prepared, tested and sufficiently close to hand to be reached by the assistant without leaving the anaesthetist's side.

Protective gloves should be worn throughout. The laryngoscope should be offered with the blade opened and correctly orientated to be grasped without adjustment. The assistant may be asked to retract the right side of the mouth or apply gentle external pressure to the larynx to improve the laryngoscopy view. *If required, laryngeal pressure and cricoid pressure must be applied in the midline, taking care not to displace the laryngeal structures laterally which can lead to distortion of the anatomy and difficulty or failure of laryngoscopy.* Similarly the tracheal tube should be handed from the right, taking care not to obstruct the laryngoscopy view with the hand or the tube. Equipment for a difficult intubation should be ready and near at hand in case they are needed.

THE RAPID SEQUENCE INDUCTION IN AN EMERGENCY CASE

Regurgitation of Gastric Contents

One of the main hazards of general anaesthesia is the vomiting or regurgitation of gastric contents into the throat, which are then aspirated into the lungs. A potentially fatal pneumonitis may follow. This was highlighted in the 1940s when Mendelson described the respiratory problems of mothers who had inhaled gastric contents at induction of anaesthesia. In the 1960s Sellick described a modified induction (the rapid sequence induction) suitable for these cases.

Normally, gastric contents are prevented from passing back up from the stomach into the throat by muscle rings in the oesophagus called the oesophageal sphincter. Protective airway reflexes stop any regurgitated material passing into the lungs. Under anaesthesia, these protective reflexes are lost. Regurgitation is uncommon because the oesophageal sphincter mechanisms remain largely intact and because preoperative fasting reduces the volume of gastric contents.

Regurgitation can occur when the oesophagel sphincter is faulty or when there is an increased volume of gastric contents. The oesophageal sphincter is abnormal in patients who are pregnant, obese or who have a family history of heartburn or hiatus hernia. A full stomach is common in emergency cases. Patients may have eaten just before admission to hospital, may have bowel obstruction or may have delayed stomach emptying because of inflammation (e.g. peritonitis), drugs (e.g. opiates) or pain. Table 3.4 lists the main situations in which a patient is at risk of regurgitation during the induction of anaesthesia.

At-risk patients may regurgitate before they are anaesthetized but they will not aspirate gastric contents because they will cough. Once intubated they may then regurgitate at any time during the operation but will not aspirate gastric contents because the cuff of the tracheal tube will prevent this. The danger period during induction of anaesthesia is therefore from loss of consciousness until the cuff of a tracheal tube is inflated in the trachea.

Table 3.4

SITUATIONS IN WHICH REGURGITATION MAY OCCUR	
Abnormal oesophageal sphincter	Pregnancy
	Hiatus hernia
	Oesophageal stricture
	Severe obesity
	History of heartburn
Full stomach	Recent solid or fluid intake
	Peritonitis of any cause
	Bowel obstruction
	Paralytic ileus – postoperative
	– drug-induced (e.g. opiates)
	Gastric carcinoma/pyloric stenosis
	Pain

Rapid Sequence Induction with Cricoid Pressure

A rapid sequence induction is modified so that the danger period is as short as possible. Instead of giving an intravenous induction agent, assessing the response and giving more if needed, a predetermined dose of induction agent is chosen and given as a rapid bolus. This is immediately followed by suxamethonium, also given rapidly. Suxamethonium is a neuromuscular blocking drug which provides rapid muscle relaxation (see below). These changes to the routine technique of induction ensure that the patient is ready to be intubated 60–90 seconds after the beginning of drug injection.

The other modification is the use of cricoid pressure (Sellick's manoeuvre) during the period from loss of consciousness until it has been verified that a tracheal tube is in position in the trachea. The cricoid cartilage is part of the larynx and is a complete cartilaginous ring; the oesophagus passes directly behind it (Fig. 3.15). Pressing firmly back on the cricoid cartilage thus compresses the oesophagus between the cricoid and the vertebral column, preventing regurgitation (Fig. 3.16).

Technique of cricoid pressure

Cricoid pressure is performed by first identifying the cricoid cartilage as the first firm prominence beneath the thyroid cartilage (the Adam's apple) and then centring it between the thumb and middle fingers of the right hand while pressing down firmly with the index finger. Good (i.e. firm) cricoid pressure sometimes pushes the neck down with the right hand while supporting the back of the neck with the left hand (bimanual cricoid pressure).

These modifications firstly shorten the period between loss of consciousness and inflation of the cuff of a tracheal tube in the trachea and secondly provide a barrier to regurgitation during this period by occluding the oesophagus with the cricoid cartilage. It is vital that cricoid pressure is continued until the position of the tracheal tube is confirmed and its cuff inflated, *even if intubation is difficult or prolonged.* Premature release of cricoid pressure may allow dangerous regurgitation.

A rapid sequence induction is thus impossible without skilled assistance. It is essential that an assistant is present who understands the technique, can apply cricoid pressure correctly and knows that it must be continued until the anaesthetist is satisfied that the tracheal tube is correctly positioned and the cuff inflated.

The precise sequence of events during a rapid sequence induction is detailed in Figure 3.17. The patient's lungs are *not* inflated with the breathing system and facemask after suxamethonium has been given, as would happen

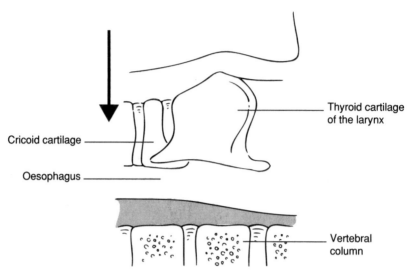

Fig. 3.15 *The larynx, oesophagus and vertebral column. Cricoid pressure is applied in the direction of the arrow*

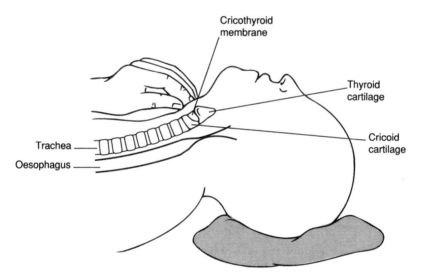

Fig. 3.16 *Technique of cricoid pressure. The cricoid cartilage is shown beneath the fingers of the left hand. The thyroid cartilage ('Adam's apple') is the protusion above it*

during a normal induction. This might disturb the oesophageal sphincter mechanism and force gas into the stomach and increase the chance of regurgitation. To prevent hypoxia during this period, the patient breathes 100% oxygen for at least 3 minutes before any drugs are injected (preoxygenation).

Suxamethonium

Suxamethonium is a depolarizing muscle relaxant and mimics the action of acetylcholine at the neuromuscular junction. It causes an initial depolarization which is clinically evident as muscle fasciculations (or twitches). This is immediately followed by profound paralysis, giving good intubating conditions more rapidly and more reliably than the non-depolarizing relaxants. Intubation is possible 50–60 seconds after doses of 1–2 mg/kg. The drug is then rapidly broken down by the enzyme plasma cholinesterase so that breathing resumes 5–10 minutes after drug injection; no reversal agent is needed.

Unfortunately, suxamethonium has numerous side-effects.

Increases in potassium concentration can be marked in patients with severe burns or recent paraplegia. Falls in heart rate are most marked with repeated injections. Muscle pains around the neck, shoulder and chest are commonest in young ambulant patients and can cause more discomfort and concern than the pain of surgery. Anaphylactoid reactions to suxamethonium can be life-threatening; it is one of the drugs most often responsible for this complication. Transient rises in intraocular and intracranial pressure can occur after suxamethonium. Malignant hyperthermia can be triggered. Finally, suxamethonium apnoea occurs in patients with an inherited deficiency of the enzyme which metabolizes suxamethonium. Treatment is by artificial ventilation with suitable sedation until recovery occurs. Investigation of the patient and family should follow.

> First ensure that suction is working and is switched on; put the suction hand piece under the patient's pillow
>
> Have a variety of tracheal tubes with introducers and bougies available
>
> Check that the patient is on a tipping trolley
>
> Attach all routine monitors
>
> Make sure the patient's head is well positioned for intubation ('sniffing' position)
>
> Preoxygenate (100% oxygen for 3 minutes)
>
> Assistant verifiess position of the cricoid cartilage
>
> Give predetermined dose of induction agent on a weight basis, followed immediately by suxamethonium (1.5 mg/kg)

Figure 3.17 Sequence of events during a rapid sequence induction with cricoid pressure. This technique requires two people: either can perform the first 6 steps; after that, the assistant's role is as detailed.

Assistant applies cricoid pressure

Wait until the patient has fasciculated (muscle tremors in response to suxamethonium) (usually 60 seconds) and then intubate

Assistant inflates cuff of tracheal tube rapidly

Check tracheal tube position (chest movement, auscultation of both lungs, capnograph trace)

Once anaesthetist is happy that tube position correct, assistant releases cricoid pressure

If cannot intubate go to failed intubation drill.

Figure 3.17 Continued

THE DIFFICULT AIRWAY AND FAILED INTUBATION DRILL

Although laryngoscopy and endotracheal intubation can be performed readily on most people, a minority of individuals provide difficulty either because of unusual anatomy or local pathology.

In 1984, two anaesthetists, Cormack and Lehane, provided a classification for difficult cases based on the view obtained at laryngoscopy.

- **Grade 1**   Most of the glottis is visible and there should be no difficulty.
- **Grade 2**   If only the posterior extremity of the glottis is visible then there may be slight difficulty. Light pressure on the larynx will nearly always bring at least the arytenoids into view if not the vocal cords.
- **Grade 3**   If no part of the glottis can be seen, only the epiglottis, then there may be fairly severe difficulty.
- **Grade 4**   If not even the epiglottis can be exposed then intubation is impossible except by alternative methods.

A number of patient factors associated with difficult intubation have been identified.

- Limited head extension
- Limited mouth opening
- Protruding upper incisors
- Distance between thyroid cartilage and chin
- Receding mandible
- Large tongue
- Obesity
- Term pregnancy

It is vital that a note is made on the patient's case record that they are a difficult intubation and why. The patient should also be alerted to tell future anaesthetists of their problem.

Failed Intubation Drill

Having a clear understanding of the management of an unexpected failed intubation is important. This is especially so when it occurs during a rapid sequence induction where there is increased risk of reflux of gastric contents. The following drill is appropriate for that situation.

1. Assistant maintains cricoid pressure.
2. Anaesthetist applies gentle positive pressure ventilation with 100% oxygen via facemask.
3. Once spontaneous respiration returns, the patient is put in the left lateral position with slight head down tilt.
4. Cricoid pressure can only be removed safely when the patient's protective reflexes have returned as the patient becomes wakeful. To maintain cricoid pressure with the patient on their side is more difficult and is maintained while the opposite hand provides support behind the patient's neck.

In some emergency situations, for example, in the presence of severe haemorrhage, the anaesthetist may decide to continue with a mask anaesthetic with spontaneous respiration. This would only occur if the patient had a good airway an the risk of aspiration was judged to be less than any delay to immediate surgery.

If failed intubation occurs during an induction with a low risk of oesophageal reflux, the anaesthetist may wish to make further attempts at intubation. For this he may wish to use a different laryngoscope blade or smaller tracheal tube. A recently introduced device is the McCoy laryngoscope blade which is shaped like a curved Macintosh blade but whose tip can be bent further using a lever device.

A most useful technique is to insert an introducer into the tracheal tube to alter the curvature of the tube. When inserting an introducer into a tube, it should be lubricated to ease removal. It is important that the tip of the introducer does not protrude beyond the distal end of the tube as this might cause damage to the larynx. Forming the introducer into a J shape is often the most helpful manoeuvre.

Some anaesthetists favour the use of a gum elastic bougie for this situation. The bougie is inserted through the larynx under direct vision. This is often easier than inserting a tracheal tube because the shape of the bougie can be altered readily and being smaller, offers a better view. Once through the larynx, the bougie can be used as a guide for a tracheal tube. The tube is passed over the bougie (railroaded) and pushed over the tongue and through the larynx blindly. This should be done gently and may require rotation of the tube to ensure smooth passage through the larynx. Once the tracheal tube is correctly positioned, the bougie is removed.

Most anaesthetic departments now have flexible fibreoptic laryngoscopes. The anaesthetist may wish to use a flexible scope to intubate the patient while they are anaesthetised. For this, a tracheal tube of appropriate size is threaded onto the scope and taped as proximally as possible. The fibrescope is then passed through the nose or mouth into the pharynx, then through the larynx under direct vision. The tracheal tube can then be advanced over the scope, using it as a guide in a similar manner as with a gum elastic bougie.

Another possible solution where the regurgitation risk is low is to use the laryngeal mask either as the definitive airway or as an introducer for a bougie, guidewire or fibreoptic laryngoscope over which an endotracheal tube is then passed.

If oxygenation of the patient cannot be maintained or the lung cannot be ventilated, a surgical airway may be needed. The simplest surgical airway is called a cricothyroid puncture. A large bore cannula is inserted through the membrane between the cricoid and thyroid cartilages and connected via an endotracheal tube connector to an anaesthetic circuit with oxygen. If available a jet ventilator can be connected to this cannula, provided another exit cannula is sited to allow expiration. There are specific kits for cricothyroid cannulation and for establishing a mini-tracheostomy using a guide wire and dilator system. In extreme cases and where the skills are available a formal tracheostomy can be carried out under local anaesthesia.

Management of the Known Difficult Intubation

The use of flexible fibreoptic laryngscopy is now the method of choice for the elective management of the known difficult intubation. Many patients who provide difficulty with intubation also provide difficulty with airway maintenance so this procedure is performed on the awake patient with topical local anaesthesia with or without sedation. The naso-tracheal route is usually preferred over the oro-tracheal as it forms a more open curve and may therefore provide a better guide.

A premedication with a drying agent to reduce salivary secretions can improve the view for this procedure. An intravenous cannula is inserted and a modest dose of a sedative may be considered if the airway is clear. The mucus membranes of the upper and lower airways must be anaesthetized with local anaesthetic. This can be applied directly to the nose with cotton wool pledgets. Further local anaesthetic administration can be applied by injecting through the open channel of the scope under direct vision. Alternatively, local anaesthetic can be applied by inhalation of nebulized 4% lignocaine from a mask. Some anaesthetists prefer to inject local anaesthetic directly to the airway by injecting through the cricothyroid membrane with a fine needle.

Once the mucus membranes are adequately numbed, the fibreoptic scope can be passed and the trachea intubated in the manner described above. During this procedure, supplemental oxygen should be administered either by mask, nasal catheter or down the channel of the laryngoscope. This method requires cooperation by the patient. This is most readily achieved if the patient is kept informed and reassured throughout.

Considerable care must be taken when handling these flexible fibreoptic instruments as they are very easily damaged and are expensive to repair. Anyone handling them should be familiar with procedures for testing, cleaning and storing them.

KEY LEARNING POINTS

1. Always be prepared for routine, difficult and failed intubations in every case.
2. Discuss the induction technique, equipment and drugs for each case with the anaesthetist in advance.
3. Ensure that an appropriate range of shapes and sizes of airway equipment are kept in stock and available.
4. Practice failed intubation drill regularly.

Further Reading

'Practical procedures in anaesthesia and critical care', Baskett PJF, Dow A, Nolan J, Maull K. Mosby, London, 1995.

Relevance

ODP Level 3   Units 4, 6, 8.

4 Induction of Regional Anaesthesia

Spinal Anaesthesia

J. H. Brown

Introduction

A spinal anaesthetic involves:

- the lower half of the body
- total loss of all sensations (pain, touch, temperature, position)
- loss of muscle power in the numb area.

In order to achieve it:

- a long fine needle is inserted in the midline in the lower back
- small volumes (1 ml to 4 ml) of local anaesthetic (LA) are injected
- the LA spreads within the fluid which surrounds the spinal cord (cerebrospinal fluid, CSF).

Other significant points are:

- the technique is fast and simple
- the area 'blocked' can extend from ribs to toes
- numbness lasts one to four hours, depending on LA used
- it is a 'sterile' procedure.

Advantages over general anaesthesia include:

- much cheaper
- avoids side-effects of general anaesthesia drugs
- patient may stay conscious and can cough – particularly when there is risk of inhaling stomach contents (emergencies, obstetrics)
- minimizes the body's 'stress response' to the pain of surgery and reduces and delays the surge of hormones which overstimulate the circulation.

Surgeons are able to operate on body structures below the umbilicus. Typical operations would include hip and knee replacement, hernia, prostate resection and Caesarean section.

Historical Development of Spinals

The technique of spinal anaesthesia evolved in Germany in the 1890s and quickly spread to Britain and the USA.
Milestones:

- 1825   Magendie described the circulation of cerebrospinal fluid (CSF)
- 1885   Corning used cocaine on spinal nerves of a dog
- 1891   Quinke and Wynter obtained cerebrospinal fluid from needles inserted into the lower back
- 1898   August Bier, a famous German surgeon, performed the first spinal. Bier used cocaine (3 ml of 0.5%) and, on one occasion, he and his assistant performed a spinal injection on each other. All seemed in order after the numbness wore off, but after 12 hours, they both developed severe headache, drowsiness and vomiting which lasted for 9 days. The first 'complications' of puncture of the dura were documented and left the way open for the development of better techniques with less risk of side-effects.
- 1943   Lignocaine was synthesized by Lofgren, the first of a new generation of safe local anaesthetics

Applied Anatomy and Physiology

There is no doubt that a skilled and informed assistant can make a significant difference to the performance and outcome of a spinal injection. This is particularly true when there are problem patients with stiff, arthritic spines or who are very overweight.

The rigid safety cell (Figs 4.1 and 4.2)

The brain is oval in shape and protected against injury by the hard bone of the skull. The spinal cord, on the other hand, is long and narrow and gives off nerve roots at regular intervals. It must also be flexible to allow the body to move easily. A complete outer protective shell would not allow this, and nature has developed a strong framework to enclose the 'cord'. It consists of 33 hollow bone blocks/vertebrae. These blocks lock into each other but can move against each other at small joints. This provides the best compromise

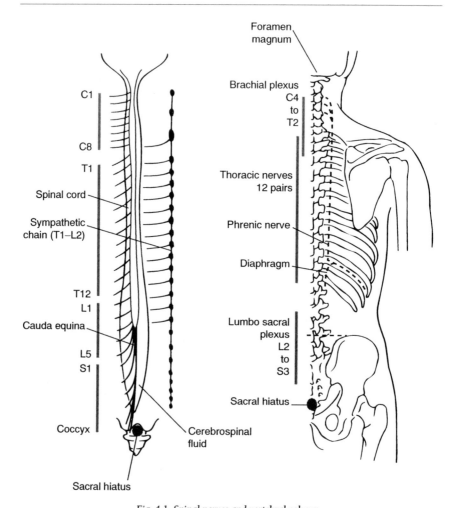

Fig. 4.1 *Spinal nerves and vertebral column*

of protection and mobility. Without the small gaps between each vertebra, injection into the spinal fluid (CSF) would not be possible.

The vertebral column comprises 7 cervical (neck), 12 thoracic (chest), 5 lumbar (lower back), 5 sacral (solid sacral bone) and 4 coccyx (remnant of evolved tail) vertebrae, making 33 bones in total.

The normal resting curves of the spinal column are of great significance when performing spinal puncture as the lumbar curve tends to reduce the gap through which the needle can pass. This 'lumbar lordosis' must be abolished as much as possible by careful positioning of the patient (flexed spine) (Figs 4.2, 4.6 and 4.7).

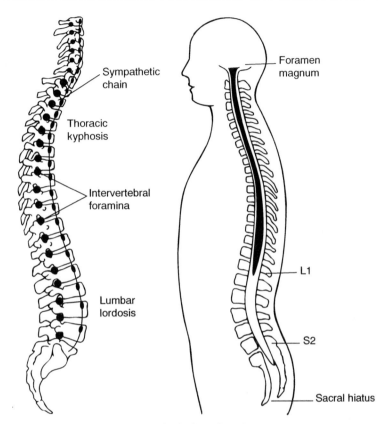

Fig. 4.2 Vertebral column, lateral view

If we consider a patient lying on his back, the lowest points of CSF are at sacral 2 and thoracic 5. This is important when considering the spread of local anaesthetic within the CSF (Figs 4.2 and 4.9).

The direction of the spinous processes are also important. In the lower lumbar area they are almost horizontal so that spinal needles are usually introduced at 90 degrees to the skin. In the thoracic area epidural needles require to be introduced at an angle (Fig. 4.8).

Spinal stability and elasticity (Fig. 4.3)

Spinal stability and elasticity is mainly due to strong ligaments which run the length of the spine:

- supraspinous ligament – joins tips of spinous processes
- interspinous ligaments – tip of introducer needle stops in it

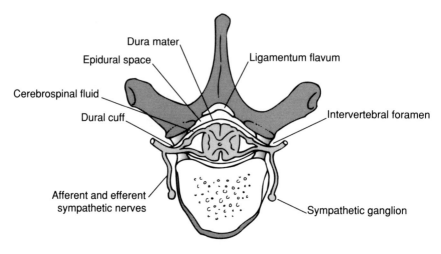

Fig. 4.3 Cross-section of thoracic vertebra

- ligamentum flavum – joins laminae of vertebrae and often causes click before needle enters epidural space
- longitudinal ligaments – related to vertebral bodies and disks, anterior and posterior.

Contents of the vertebral canal (Figs 4.1 and 4.3)

The vertebral canal extends from the base of the skull (foramen magnum) to the sacral hiatus (a small depression which can be felt between the sacrum and the coccyx at the base of the spine). It contains:

1. Spinal cord – this extends from the foramen magnum to the upper border of the second lumbar vertebra. It is approximately 45 cm long. Below the lumbar 2 level there are only individual nerve fibres which descend vertically to their exit points (foramina) and are termed the cauda equina.
2. Fibrous sheaths – the dura mater forms a tubular sheath from foramen magnum to lower border of 2nd sacral vertebra. The arachnoid mater (like a spider's web) is a thin layer attached to the inside of the dura. The CSF circulates inside the sac formed by the dura/arachnoid.
3. Subarachnoid space – contains spinal cord, nerve fibres and CSF. Local anaesthetics injected into this space can diffuse as far as the brain itself if a sufficient amount is introduced.
4. Extradural space – otherwise known as peri- and epi-dural space (the space outside the dura). Contains fat, blood vessels and fibrous tissue. At

the intervertebral foramina it communicates with the paravertebral space which is close to the chest cavity. Thus the pressure inside the chest or the abdomen will have an effect on extradural pressure. The space stretches from the foramen magnum to the sacral hiatus.

5. Spinal nerves – the spinal cord is segmentalized by 31 pairs of symmetrically arranged nerves. There are 8 cervical, 12 thoracic, 5 lumbar, 5 sacral and 1 coccygeal. The anterior and posterior nerve roots unite just before they leave the extradural space at the intervertebral foramina.

6. Cerebrospinal fluid (CSF):
   - clear fluid containing glucose, protein and salt
   - produced inside brain – 150 ml per day
   - total volume is approximately 130 ml, of which 35 ml is in spinal canal
   - pressure depends on pressure inside skull.
   - The specific gravity (SG), the relative heaviness compared to water (1000), of CSF is around 1003, and this has led to local anaesthetics being formulated in the following ways: hypobaric, lighter than CSF and tends to rise as it disperses; hyperbaric, heavier than CSF and tends to sink. Glucose is used to increase the SG of the solution (1013); isobaric, same SG as CSF and spread depends upon other factors.

Respiratory mechanics

Normal breathing depends on two groups of muscles with completely different nerve supply. Most important is the diaphragm, supplied by the phrenic nerve from cervical 3, 4, 5 roots. Less important are the intercostals, supplied from 12 pairs of thoracic nerves.

The diaphragm separates the chest contents from the abdominal contents. The intercostal muscles are found between the ribs.

Normal spinal blockade frequently involves some of the lower thoracic nerves but this has minimal effect on breathing as the diaphragm is functioning. If too much local anaesthetic is injected and the height of block reaches the mid cervical level, artificial ventilation of the lungs will be required because the diaphragm and intercostal muscles will be paralysed.

The sympathetic nervous system (Figs 4.1–4.3)

A conscious individual is aware of the functioning of the sensory/motor nerves. For instance, if a hand is put into very hot water it takes a fraction of a second for this to be appreciated and then motor nerves are used to contract muscles which will withdraw the hand.

The body also possesses an autonomic or vegetative nervous system which usually functions automatically to control processes which we are not normally aware of, such as digestion, secretions from glands, heart rate and circulation of blood to various organs. Normally there is a balance between two opposing autonomic systems:

Parasympathetic	*Sympathetic*
(rest and rebuild tissues)	(defence, ready for action)
stimulates digestion	stops digestion
lowers heart rate	increases heart rate
lowers blood pressure	increases blood pressure

The sympathetic system has its origin in nerves which leave the spinal cord with the anterior nerve roots from thoracic 1 to lumbar 2 level. The small fibres run to the ganglia in the sympathetic chains which lie on either side of the thoracic and lumbar vertebral bodies. From there small fibres run to the heart, lungs and abdominal viscera. Also they surround blood vessels.

The extent of the 'sympathetic block' which accompanies spinals and epidurals is associated with the extent to which the blood pressure falls.

Preparation for Induction of Spinal Anaesthesia

Preparation of patient

It is important to remember that the basic rules which apply for general anaesthesia also apply for regional techniques. If spinal blockade is impossible to perform, or fails, then a general anaesthetic may be required. The patient must be fasting and must also have received proper assessment and explanation.

The premedication visit is the time when the anaesthetist gives serious consideration to the type of anaesthesia which will best suit an individual patient. Numerous factors must be considered before intradural blockade is selected as the method of choice for that patient.

Suitability of patient?

The technique is ideal for fit patients who are afraid of being 'put to sleep' perhaps because of unpleasant associations with vets putting animals down. It allows large, muscular patients who perhaps drink too much alcohol to avoid large doses of anaesthetic drugs.

Special indications:

- higher risk patients (medical problem or previous drug reaction)
- full stomach (trauma or surgical emergency)

- disease of airways and lungs
- diabetic patients
- previous history of prolonged vomiting after general anaesthetic.

Once the decision for spinal blockade is made, certain considerations become more important in comparison with general anaesthesia.

The patient will be aware of what is happening during the spinal injection and will be able to cooperate better if there has been careful explanation of positioning and physical sensations as block progresses.

The patient may worry about what happens if the block wears off during surgery. It must be made clear that if this very unlikely event occurs a general anaesthetic would normally be given immediately.

Major contraindications to spinal anaesthesia:

- refusal of patient
- disorders of blood clotting and patients on anti-clotting drugs
- significant chronic disease of nervous system
- infection at area of injection or generalized body sepsis
- shock – from blood loss or dehydration
- significant disease of heart and circulation, for example recent heart attack,

In the past there has been a tendency for other doctors to blame 'the spinal' if a chronic disease of muscle or nervous tissue flares up in the postoperative period. More importantly, very unfit patients may be put at considerable risk if a spinal block extends too far or if the blood pressure falls suddenly. Having said this, spinal anaesthesia performed by a skilled anaesthetist is a very safe procedure. It has stood the test of time and is still the most widely used form of central nerve blockade.

Spinal anaesthesia may be difficult in the following situations:

- obvious deformity or stiffness of vertebral column
- history of recurring severe headache or low backache
- high-risk patients if anaesthetist is inexperienced
- disc prolapse (slipped disc)
- spinal metastases (invasion of spinal bones by cancer)
- osteoporosis (thinning of the bones)

Suitability of operation?

Spinal anaesthesia is best for operations below the umbilicus.

If the surgery will involve pulling on the peritoneum, for example Caesarean section or appendix, the anaesthetist will aim at a high block to the thoracic 4/5 dermatomal level. Otherwise the patient will become distressed and perhaps vomit.

The predicted duration of surgery also plays a part in the decision. It is not sensible to use spinals for very short operations if a general anaesthetic is not contraindicated. Equally the spinal may wear off if the duration is greater than 3 to 4 hours.

Table 4.4

HOW HIGH SHOULD THE BLOCK GO?		
OPERATION	**HEIGHT**	**DERMATOME**
Major abdominal, Caesarean section	Nipple line	Thoracic 4
Pelvis gynaecology, Appendix	Xiphoid	Thoracic 6
Prostate, hip surgery	Umbilicus	Thoracic 10
Upper, leg, lower leg amputation	Groin	Lumbar 1
Knee and below	Thigh	Lumbar 2/3
Haemorrhoids	Perineum	Sacral 2/5

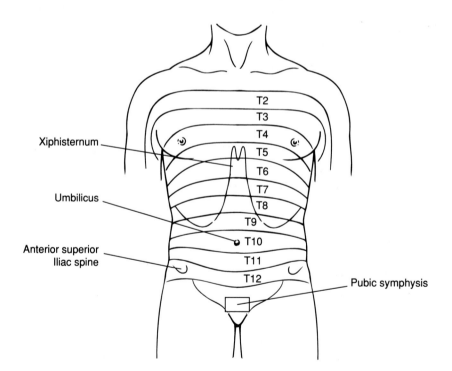

Fig. 4.4 Anterior representation of dermatomes of thoracic nerves

An anaesthetic assistant must be very careful if he or she attempts to discuss the conduct of the 'spinal' with the patient preoperatively. The anaesthetist may well have given the patient a detailed explanation, and a conflicting description of injection position or sensations which will be experienced as the blockade progresses will only serve to shake the patient's confidence.

Preparation of anaesthetic room and theatre

General preparations:

- set up for general anaesthesia (mask, airways, intubation equipment, suction apparatus)
- check supply of gases
- lay out all drugs required for general anaesthesia
- prepare intravenous infusion (1 litre Ringer lactate or 0.9% saline)
- lay out larger size cannula (16G or 14G)
- monitoring (ECG, blood pressure and oximetry)
- tipping trolley with firm brakes
- light plastic oxygen mask with tubing
- height-adjustable stools; one for anaesthetist and one for feet of sitting patient

Specific preparations:

1. Mobile trolley on which packs can be opened. Shelf beneath on which all sterile packs, needles and ampoules can be laid out ready for opening.
2. Gloves and gown for the anaesthetist.
3. Basic sterile pack which is opened out first using scrupulous aseptic technique. It could be a basic minor-op pack from theatre sterile supply unit or a compact, disposable, single-use commercial pack. A typical single-use pack contains:
   - spinal needle
   - introducer for spinal needle
   - large swab
   - smaller swabs or sponges for washing back
   - small galley pot to hold antiseptic solution
   - sponge holder or forceps (plastic)
   - 25G needle for skin infiltration
   - 16G or 18G needle for drawing up solutions
   - small filter to stop glass fragments and bacteria entering syringe
   - syringes (2 ml) for skin infiltration and 5 ml for spinal injection.

4. Spinal needles (Fig. 4.5), steel of thickness 22G to 29G and 9 cm (3.5 inches) long. They contain a central stilette which is kept in place until needle is in subarachnoid space. This is so that no particles of skin contaminate the CSF. An introducer needle, through which the spinal needle is inserted, is also used to minimize contamination. The risk of postspinal headache is lessened by using narrower needles (usually 24 to 26G). Many anaesthetists feel that the relatively blunt pencil-point needles (Whitacre or Sprotte) with side openings reduce the incidence of headache even further.

5. Local anaesthetic agents – it would be possible to use many agents but, in practice, only bupivacaine is freely available. Lignocaine is used, but much less frequently, and amethocaine can be obtained by special arrangement.

Bupivacaine (Marcain) – isobaric 0.5% and 0.75% available, hyperbaric 0.5% in 8% Glucose (4 ml ampoule).
● Hyperbaric – fixation time, 10 to 30 minutes; SG, 1013; duration, 160 minutes.
● Isobaric – more localized effect with longer duration. Good for hip operations in elderly as patient can lie on good side during injection.

Lignocaine (Xylocain) – 2% preservative and glucose free, 5% hyperbaric in 7.5% glucose (2 ml ampoule).

Amethocaine (Tetracaine, Pantocaine) – prepared as dried powder in 20 mg ampoules or as 1% solution in 2 ml ampoules. Not commonly used.

6. Drugs: sedation – midazolam or anaesthetist's preference; emergency – atropine, vasoconstrictors (ephedrine, methoxamine).

7. Have selection of music cassettes, player and earphones available. Check patient's preference.

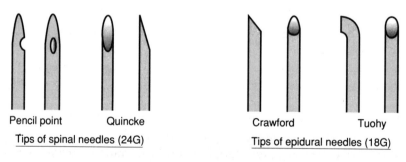

Pencil point   Quincke   Crawford   Tuohy
Tips of spinal needles (24G)   Tips of epidural needles (18G)

Fig. 4.5 Tips of spinal and epidural needles

The safe conduct of spinal anaesthesia

A skilled assistant has a large part to play in the practicalities of performing the 'block'. Should there be a 'difficult' back, the assistant with sound knowledge of patient positioning can make things much easier for the anaesthetist, often without being asked.

Psychology

Get to know your anaesthetist. if the anaesthetist perceives that the proper preparations have been made and that any special materials that he requires are ready (correct glove size, correct needle type) he will have great confidence in the assistant and will be more likely to perform a good block.

Get to know the patient. If you can visit the patient preoperatively so much the better. If not, it is important to notice as quickly as possible if the patient is very anxious. He/she may be remaining awake for the procedure and you may have to chat to the patient for several hours. You can strike up a rapport while going through the necessary checking procedures of name, operation site, etc.

Preliminaries in anaesthetic room

Set up routine monitoring. Blood pressure cuff, ECG and oximeter probe. Take one control blood pressure and then set automatic BP cuff to 'standby'. It will not be required until after the spinal injection. Lay out anaesthetic record so that control values may be entered. The assistant should check the vital signs when the anaesthetist is preoccupied with the procedure by observing the ECG, NIBP, and Sp O_2 readings.

Prepare intravenous infusion of crystalloid (Ringer's lactate). A 14G or 16G cannula should be used as a sudden fall in blood pressure may require *rapid* infusion.

Positioning the patient (Figs 4.6 and 4.7)

Depending on the height of block required and the fitness of the patient the anaesthetist will then decide on the position for injection. Instructions and explanation must be given to the patient before any move is attempted.

Lying on side. This is easily tolerated by most patients and tends to antagonize any fall in blood pressure after the injection. The patient should slide over until his back is just at the edge of the trolley. He is then told to curve his back 'like a cat' by pulling knees up to chest and also flexing the head to make the chin touch the upper sternum. This will 'open the back' (Fig 4.6a) and will allow most injections to be done. If the anaesthetist is having trouble

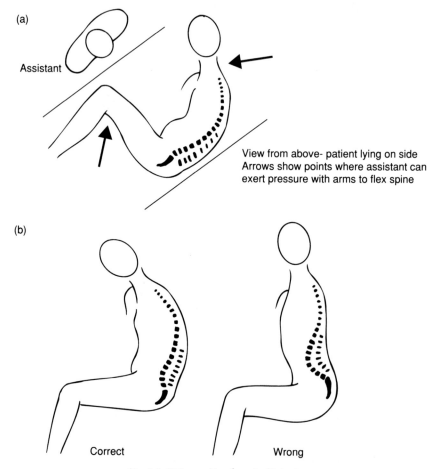

(a)

Assistant

View from above- patient lying on side
Arrows show points where assistant can
exert pressure with arms to flex spine

(b)

Correct   Wrong

Fig. 4.6 Sitting position for spinal injection

locating the subarachnoid space (elderly, calcified spine, obesity) the assistant
can exert slight pressure from an arm behind the neck and the other behind
the knees to further flex the lumbar spine.

Sitting position. Easier to perform the injection and therefore good position
for inexperienced anaesthetists. The patient has legs over edge of trolley with
feet on height-adjustable stool. A pillow is put on patients' knees and the
patient told to rest elbows on pillow and lean slightly forward. The patient is
supported at all times by the assistant to prevent forward or lateral falling
(Fig. 4.6b).

Other positions such as lying on stomach for low approach to lumbar
5/sacral 1 interspace have been used in the past, but are very rarely used today.

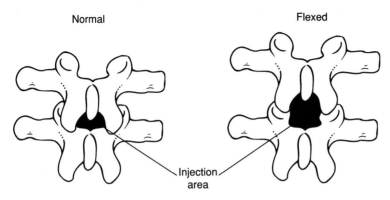

Fig. 4.7 View from behind with lumbar spine flexion

Marking the back

It is important that the anaesthetist knows exactly the location of the lumbar 3/4 interspace. This is done once the patient is positioned by considering a line between the iliac crests. This crosses the spine of the L4 vertebra or the L4/L5 space. A marker pen is then used (Fig. 4.1).

Disinfection

The anaesthetist should wear appropriate theatre hat, mask and sterile gloves and sit on a stool behind the patient. The assistant must take great care to maintain sterility when opening out sterile packs, ampoules, etc.

Location of subarachnoid space (Figs 4.3 and 4.8)

A small bleb of local anaesthetic is first raised over the chosen interspace using a 25G needle. Through this 1 to 2 ml of 1% lignocaine can be injected into subcutaneous area and interspinous ligament. The larger introducer is then inserted into the interspinous ligament. The spinal needle with its central stilette is firmly pushed through it until the anaesthetist senses that tissue resistance is less. When the central spinal needle stilete is removed CSF should flash back into the plastic chamber or drop from a metal hub. The needle is in the correct place and the injection can be given.

Control of spread of nerve block

An experienced anaesthetist knows that the extent of spread of anaesthesia depends on numerous factors. Certain of these can be controlled in a practical way so that the necessary degree of anaesthesia is obtained.

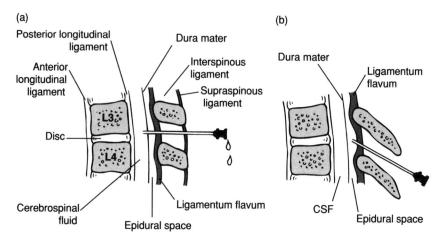

Fig. 4.8 (a) Midline section (lumbar), spinal injection. (b) Thoracic approach, epidural injection

1. Preinjection patient position. This makes use of the specific gravity of the injected solution. If high block with hyperbaric solution is desired the patient should be lying on his side while for a saddle block of the perineum the sitting position is required. Remember that the preinjection position is also the first postinjection position as it takes time to remove the needle, attach a dressing and move the patient.

2. Patient factors: age, height, weight, length of back. The anaesthetist may inject more solution if X-rays and other factors indicate a long back, a wide vertebral canal and a larger spinal volume of CSF. If the patient is old, frail or very ill or if pregnant, the volume injected may be reduced.

3. Injection Factors:
   - interspace through which injection is given
     – L2/3 for abdominal procedures
     – L3/4 for pelvis and legs
     – L4/5 for saddle block of perineum
   - volume of local anaesthetic
   - concentration of local anaesthetic
   - force and rate of injection
   - specific gravity of local anaesthetic
   - barbotage (mixing with CSF): at two or three stages during the injection CSF is sucked back (0.5 to 1 ml) and allowed to mix with syringe contents.

4. Postinjection patient position (Fig. 4.9). No pronounced effect is seen

Spread T 10–S 5

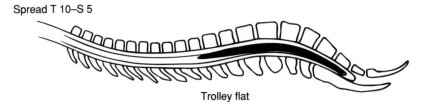

Trolley flat

Spread T 5–S 5

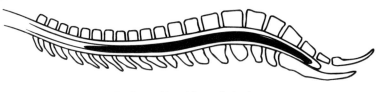

Trolley 15° headdown tilt 3 minutes

Injection – lying on side L3/4
Volume – 3ml hyperbaric
Post injection position – lying on back

Fig. 4.9 Effects of postinjection positioning on height of blockade

with isobaric LA. With hyperbaric and hypobaric LA the patient may be put into a 15° head down or head up tilt for a few minutes post injection. The patient may either be kept in a lateral position or moved onto their back.

Assessment of the progress of the blockade

The narrowest nerves are affected first and the block quickly progresses to the largest motor nerve fibres which supply muscles. Ultimately the muscles are relaxed and the patient loses all power. The blocked area spreads from the legs upwards over the stomach.

The skin dermatomal level reached by the block may be estimated using a swab containing some melting ice. It is unnecessary to continually use a sharp needle tip except for assessment of final height of block. There is a certain fixation time until the block is complete (approximately 5 min for lignocaine and 10–30 min for bupivacaine) and during this period the patient may say that the lower limbs or bottom feel 'warm' or 'tingly'. There may be pins and needles sensation and the limbs may feel heavy. Ultimately the patient notices that the legs cannot be moved and that a feeling of numbness is spreading onto the abdomen.

It is important that patients undergoing a saddle block of the perineum know that the legs may not go numb.

Management during the immediate postinjection phase

It is critical that the patient is carefully observed during this period. Trends in heart rate and blood pressure coupled with changes in patient behaviour will permit side-effects and complications to be detected early and suitable measures to be taken.

1. Measure pulse and blood pressure every minute and enter on record.
2. Assess ascent of block with cold stimulation of skin.
3. Observe patient – note pallor, restlessness, retching. The patient may say:
   'I feel funny'
   'I feel ill'
   'I think I am going to be sick'
   'I can't breathe properly'.

Check again that all resuscitation equipment and drugs are to hand. The patient may also be taking note of what you are doing so remember the three Cs – calmness, confidence, control.

Management during the operation

1. *Never leave the patient alone.* Someone should stay near the patient's head at all times to provide reassurance and explanation.
2. Ensure that exactly the same physiological monitoring is applied as if general anaesthesia had been used.
3. Blood pressure continues to be important, especially for patients with hypertension and poor circulation to heart and brain. Drugs which increase blood pressure may be required to raise blood pressure to a level the anaesthetist considers safe.
4. Sedation may or may not be necessary. If the patient is calm it is nice to offer music from a cassette player and to have a selection of musical styles available. Make sure the earphones are comfortable and that the volume is adjusted to the patient's preference.
5. Oxygen via a light plastic mask (Hudson) is always a good idea. It may even be combined with nitrous oxide (25 to 40%) to provide a small degree of analgesia for the back, shoulders and arms which may ache from being in a fixed position for several hours.

Normal side-effects of spinal blockade

Heart and circulation – low block, slight fall in blood pressure; high block, large fall in blood pressure, heart rate falls.

Respiratory – breathing tends to become slow and shallow. The ability to breathe in depends on the 5th to 9th intercostal nerves and on the diaphragm supplied by the phrenic nerves (cervical 3, 4, 5). There is usually no problem and oxygen saturation monitoring will confirm that all is well.

Gastrointestinal – the bowel becomes contracted, which has advantages for surgery on the gut itself. Nausea and vomiting may occur, caused mainly by low blood pressure (below 80 systolic usually), pulling on peritoneum (hernia or appendix), psychological reaction (anxiety, hysteria).

Central nervous system – the amount of electrical information reaching the brain is reduced and the patient may become drowsy. If blood pressure is low and too little oxygen is being given the patient may become agitated.

Endocrine – normal response of the adrenal glands to pain is delayed. There is no outpouring of hormones and diabetic patients do not tend to be made worse. The 'stress response' normally does occur under general anaesthesia.

Kidneys – low blood pressure will reduce production of urine by reducing the perfusion of the renal glomeruli.

Body temperature – adrenal gland secretions are depressed so metabolism and heat production decrease. Vasodilatation of skin allows increased rate of heat loss from large body surface. This is important for long operations (2–3 hours).

Management is by heated water blanket under patient, 'space' blanket under drapes, warmer for I/V fluids, raise theatre temperature, prewarm bed in recovery room.

Complications of spinal anaesthesia

Early complications will require the assistant to act quickly and efficiently.

Severe and rapid fall in blood pressure – the causes have already been described. It is usually accompanied by slowing of heart rate, nausea and obvious patient upset. Below 80 mmHg treatment is usually required. It usually occurs within 5 min of injection but can occur after up to 20 min. It is more likely in unfit and already shocked patients (trauma, dehydration).

Treatment is oxygen via mask (Hudson), head down tilt of trolley, rapid intravenous infusion – up to 1 litre, vasopressor drugs (ephedrine, methoxamine), atropine to increase heart rate.

Total spinal – characterized by initial patient restlessness, blood pressure suddenly unrecordable, respiration stops, pupils increase in size, patient becomes unconscious.

A total spinal is a *real* crisis and demands immediate attention. *Do not panic.*

Management is to ventilate patient with 100% oxygen, have equipment ready for intubation, lift legs up to increase central blood volume, treat low blood pressure as above. The respiratory paralysis can last for several hours and artificial ventilation will be required.

Delayed complications occur from hours to days after the spinal and should not make any demands on the assistant. Detailed description of symptoms and management may be obtained from standard anaesthetic textbooks.

- Headache – may be severe and prolonged. Commoner in young people.
- Backache – this is a common complaint and it is also common after general anaesthesia. Cause is uncertain.
- Urinary retention – this is relatively frequent (14–37%) and may have several causes: bladder nerves are sacral 2, 3, 4 and recover function late, it is often difficult to pass water when lying supine, fluid given to maintain blood pressure causes the bladder to distend when sensations absent. If no urine is passed after 4 hours or more a catheter may be inserted.
- Neurological – extremely rare. Infection or mistaken injection of wrong substances may result in pain, numbness, muscle weakness and possibly bladder and bowel disturbances. Paraplegia has occurred in very few cases.

EPIDURAL ANAESTHESIA

J. H. Brown

Introduction

In the early 1940s Massey Dawkins performed the first epidural block in Britain. Then, in 1945, Tuohy developed his famous needle with the curved tip which was capable of placing a catheter in the epidural space. The technique was made popular in the 1970s as a method of providing 'painless labour' during childbirth.

Epidural and spinal anaesthesia have so many similarities that it is almost impossible to describe one without reference to the other. The reader is therefore encouraged to first of all read the previous section on spinal anaesthesia. The techniques have two major differences:

- the epidural space extends from the base of the skull to the sacral hiatus. It is possible to perform an injection anywhere along it from the neck to the sacrum. A spinal/intradural injection must be performed in the lower lumbar area so as not to damage the spinal cord.

- the quality of nerve blockade is not as intense as with spinals. The small pain fibres are always blocked but larger nerves such as touch, position sense, and motor to muscles are frequently not blocked.

Applied Anatomy and Physiology (Figs 4.1 and 4.3)

The extradural space is the gap between the tough dural sheath and the bones and ligaments of the vertebral column. It is triangular in shape. It extends further than the dura and opens at the sacral hiatus. Thus, large volumes of local anaesthetic injected at the sacral hiatus (caudal block) can progress a considerable way to the epidural space, even to the lower chest level.

The ligamentum flavum is of great importance as it is relatively thick and rich in elastic fibres. The sudden loss of resistance as the epidural needle emerges from it into the epidural space is the key to safe injection with avoidance of dural puncture.

The epidural space contains loose connective tissue, fat, arteries, veins and lymph vessels. The spinal nerve roots are in the lateral parts of the epidural triangle before they enter the intervertebral foramina.

Whilst a needle may be inserted into the space throughout its length, it is safest and simplest in the lumbar area as the spinal processes are horizontal and the space is also at its widest. In the mid thorax the spines are at a significant downward slant and the space is much narrower – altogether more difficult to locate (Fig. 4.8).

Comparison of Epidural and Spinal (Intradural) Blockade

General similarities

The indications, contraindications and preparations for epidural injection are broadly similar to those for spinal injection. It is suitable for as wide a variety of operations and it has the same site of action and similar side-effect profile.

Volume and toxicity

Whereas spinals require less that 3 ml of solution, epidurals may require up to 20 ml for extensive block as the local anaesthetic 'leaks' out through the intervertebral foramina. The extent of block is not as easy to predict or control and certain other side-effects are possible: (1) toxic reaction from high plasma levels, and (2) sudden collapse of blood pressure and circulation if accidental injection into epidural blood vessel.

Time course

The local anaesthetic has to penetrate the thick dural cuff round the mixed nerves and the 'onset' time is therefore much longer than with spinal.

Combinations with general anaesthesia

The quality of block is not as complete as with spinals, so a light general anaesthetic is often combined with the epidural. For major surgery the epidural is the analgesic component of 'balanced anaesthesia', where it also contributes a degree of muscle relaxation.

Headache

If the epidural is properly executed there is no risk of post injection headache. Unfortunately, epidural needles are much larger than spinal (16G versus 25G) and accidental dural puncture has a high incidence of severe headache due to leakage of cerebrospinal fluid.

Special therapeutic uses of epidural

- Obstetrics – pain relief in labour, Caesarean section
- Postoperative pain relief – usually with catheter
- Pain relief – chest injuries (fractured ribs)
              – stones in kidneys and gall bladder ducts
              – chronic pain (lower back common)
              – cancer pain (infusions via indwelling catheter)

Preparation for Induction of Extradural Blockade

General preparations

Most of the considerations applied to intradural block also apply to epidural. Detailed assessment of patient position is not so important, as the epidural needle/catheters may be inserted as the appropriate level for surgery (thoracic included) and are more frequently combined with general anaesthesia.

It is also important to explain to the patient that it may only be pain fibres which are blocked and that feelings of touch and movement do not indicate that the block has failed. It is even more important to assure the patient that if uncomfortable sensations do occur, adequate sedation/general anaesthesia will be given immediately.

Specific preparations

Epidural needles (Fig. 4.5).

- Tuohy. The standard needle used. It is 8 cm long with the shaft graduated in centimetres. Width is 16G or 18G and it has a closely fitting stilette inside it to add rigidity to the relatively thin-walled shaft. The point is rounded and blunt with the outlet shaped to allow a plastic catheter to emerge at an angle of 20°. A longer version is available for larger patients.
- Crawford. Not so common and has short normal level. Catheter passes easily but needle must enter epidural space at an angle if catheter is not to stick against the dura. It is therefore better when paramedian approach is used.

Single use packs. These are used by most anaesthetists as they are of very high quality with guaranteed sterility. The needles, catheters and filter fit perfectly together. A typical set will contain:

- 1 epidural needle
- 1 25G needle for skin infiltration
- 1 25G needle for deeper infiltration
- 1 drawing up needle with filter
- 1 10ml 'loss of resistance' device
- 1 20ml syringe for local anaesthetic solution
- 1 5ml syringe for infiltration
- adhesive drape with central opening
- large and small swabs, sponge holder and galley pot for antiseptic.

Optional:
- graduated catheter with blind-ended tip
- filter for continuous infusion or repeat injections.

Local anaesthetic agents. Lignocaine – 1% gives good analgesia but 2% necessary if muscle relaxation is required. It has a short 'onset' time (6 min) but the effects are certainly wearing off after 2 hours. Prilocaine – available usually as 2% solution. Has slightly longer 'onset' time and duration of action than lignocaine. Bupivacaine – most commonly used and available as 0.25%, 0.5% and 0.75% solutions. It is relatively slow to have effect but has long duration of action (4–6 hours). Adrenaline 1/200,000 may be added to these agents to produce faster onset and longer duration of action. It slows the absorption of local into epidural blood vessels.

The Safe Conduct of Epidural Anaesthesia

The preparations, positioning and disinfection procedures for epidural anaesthesia are broadly similar to those for spinal anaesthesia, but there are certain obvious differences in technique. After subcutaneous infiltration at the appropriate interspace a small blade is often used to make a clean skin incision 4 mm or so in length, through which the epidural needle is inserted until it is firmly located in the interspinous ligament. This is so that skin particles are not transported on the needle tip into the epidural space.

Location of epidural space

Loss of resistance technique. Once the Tuohy needle is in the interspinous ligament the central stilette is removed and a 10 ml loss of resistance device containing either air or saline is attached. The anaesthetist uses one hand to advance the needle while the other exerts a constant pressure on the syringe plunger. When the ligamentum flavum is reached there is great resistance to injection, but as soon as the ligament is pierced the resistance disappears. Once it is certain that no CSF or blood can be aspirated through the needle, then the 'test' dose of local anaesthesia may be injected.

Other techniques. There are several of these including use of small spring loaded syringes or air-filled balloons, but the most used has been the 'hanging drop' method. A drop of saline is placed in the hub of the advancing needle. When the tip is in the epidural space the negative pressure sucks the drop into the needle.

It is important that the patient does not make sudden movements as the needle is advancing. The assistant must maintain the patient carefully in the chosen position, giving reassurance if necessary.

Insertion of catheter

The catheter has a blocked off tip, with 3 or more side holes in the first 2 cm. It therefore must be inserted 3 to 4 cm into space.

The catheter is never pulled through the needle as it may be sheared through by the sharp edge at the curve of the Tuohy needle tip. A small length of catheter would then be lost in the epidural space.

The anaesthetist takes great care to avoid kinking the catheter as it is fixed to the back with adhesive tape. It is usually then led up over the shoulder. The filter attached to the end rests on the pillow next to the patient's head.

The 'test' dose

Most anaesthetists give a small injection of local through the catheter and, if no signs of spinal blockade are present after a few minutes, the full calculated volume of solution is injected. Catheters have also been known to perforate the dura and a first 'test dose' is also given via the catheter.

Control of spread of epidural blockade

Prediction is less easy than with spinal as the injection volume must be estimated and several factors must be taken into account. Specific gravity is irrelevant. On average, 1.5 ml of local is injected per dermatomal segment to be blocked.

Assessment of the progress of the blockade

Positioning of the patient after injection has very little influence on spread of blockade (unlike spinal). A needle, ice cube or skin pinch may be used to map the areas of skin insensitive to sharp pain or cold (touch sensation may be intact).

The monitoring, management and normal side-effects of epidural block are to all intents and purposes identical to spinal anaesthesia. However, blood pressure should not fall suddenly, and effects on respiratory muscles are much less marked. If a general anaesthetic is to be given in addition to the epidural it is usual for the anaesthetist to wait until the epidural is obviously starting to work. During and after induction of the GA it is even more important to monitor blood pressure.

Complications of Extradural Blockade

These are similar to those for spinal but certain accidental and unwanted sequelae are particular to epidural techniques.

Early: immediate to 60 minutes

Dural puncture – this is associated with unpleasant headache in 70% of cases. When it occurs it may be possible for the anaesthetist to convert to spinal anaesthesia, or withdraw the needle and insert an epidural catheter at a segment above or below the perforation. An epidural catheter may also perforate the dura and most anaesthetists check for aspiration of CSF through the catheter before local is injected. The headache may be severe with dizziness, vomiting and black, sunken eyes.

Treatment is flat in bed (prone position best), analgesics, high oral fluid intake, epidural infusion of saline (60 ml per hour), epidural blood patch (if severe and persistent). Some favour early blood patch treatment. This involves taking 0.25–0.5 ml/kg of the patient's own venous blood under aseptic conditions and injecting it via an epidural needle into the epidural space.

This forms a clot which seals the hole in the dura and the headache often immediately disappears.

Accidental subarachnoid injection – may result in a 'total spinal' block. Signs and management are as described above. A true 'life and death' crisis.

Massive epidural block – due to excessive spread and represents a complete miscalculation by the anaesthetist of factors such as age or diabetes. It may present just like a 'total spinal' and has similar management.

Puncture of epidural vein – associated with late pregnancy and also with needle direction slightly off the midline. Great care is taken not to thread a catheter up an epidural vein. Injection into a vein will result in a major and life threatening 'toxic reaction'.

Late: hours to days (assistant will not normally be involved)

Further information on urine retention, headache and neurological complications may be found in any standard anaesthetic textbook.

Special Techniques

Caudal block

Caudal block produces excellent blockade of the sacral nerves. Thus it is useful for operations in the perineal area, for example anus (haemorrhoids), rectum, penis (circumcision), urethra (cystoscopy) and vagina (childbirth).

Applied anatomy (Figs 4.1, 4.2 and 4.10). The sacrum is the curved posterior wall of the pelvis and results from the fusion of the 5 sacral vertebrae. There

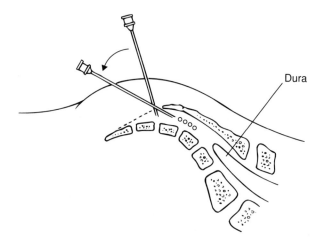

Dura

Fig. 4.10 Caudal injection with patient face down

is considerable variation in the size and shape of the sacral hiatus, but it is usually triangular and approximately 16 mm wide by 20 mm in height. The hiatus is covered by the sacrococcygeal ligament which is punctured to enter the canal. The lower part of the canal contains sacral and coccygeal nerve roots, fat, connective tissue and blood vessels. The subarachnoid space ends in adults at S2 level.

Particular advantages:

- low risk of dural puncture
- low volume, low toxicity, fall in blood pressure unlikely
- maintains power and sensation in abdomen and legs.

The contraindications are as for spinal and epidural, especially with regard to localized infection.

Preparations. Similar considerations to epidural anaesthesia apply to the caudal approach with respect to concentrations and volumes of solution. There are special caudal needles but many anaesthetists use ordinary disposable hypodermic needles. A catheter may be inserted if prolonged analgesia is required.

Position. Two main positions – lying face down (prone) or on side with knees drawn up. Prone, a pillow under hips with legs slightly apart and feet turned to each other. A swab is placed between the buttocks so that antiseptic solution cannot run down over anus and genitals (can irritate and 'burn'). The site of injection is disinfected, covered with a drape with central opening, and the site infiltrated with local. The sacrococcygeal ligament is pierced at 90° and the needle then moved through 45° before it is advanced into the canal (Fig. 4.10).

Thoracic epidural (Figs 4.3 and 4.8b)

The practical problems have already been described above. It is without doubt more difficult and risky than the lumbar approach and only skilled anaesthetists should attempt it. It has particular advantages in that the lower half of the body is not affected by sensory or motor block. If a catheter is inserted, excellent analgesia may be extended into the postoperative phase.

Epidural opioids

The effect of epidural opioids is due to the blockade of morphine-type receptors in the spinal cord. Sympathetic nerves, motor, touch and so on are unaffected. Compared to oral or intramuscular doses of opioid, the quality of analgesia is better and the central side-effects are less. Intermittent injections or slow infusions are given via a catheter.

There are two main indications:

- postoperative pain relief
- management of chronic cancer pain.
  Side-effects – these are less frequent than after oral ingestion:

- nausea and vomiting
- constipation
- respiratory depression
- retention of urine
- itching.

The respiratory depression may be early or delayed and can result from accidental subarachnoid injection. The opioids reach the respiratory centre in the midbrain. If severe, naloxone will be necessary.

Postoperative pain relief with epidural opioids requires careful observation particularly of respiratory function.

Combined spinal and epidural

This applies mainly in obstetrics where special techniques have been developed to allow spinal blockade to be accomplished via a very fine (26G) needle inserted through a Tuohy needle. A catheter may also be inserted into the epidural space.

Nerve Block Procedure

K. M. Rogers

Nerve blocks are performed to anaesthetize specific isolated areas of the body for surgery, but as they may provide up to 8 hours pain relief after surgery, the postoperative period is made much more comfortable for the patient with less requirement for analgesics such as morphine, and less attention by nursing staff. If no general anaesthetic has been employed then the patients do not need a protracted stay in the recovery area and can eat or drink soon after their return to the ward.

It is important that the patient is in the theatre area where they are to receive their block at least one hour before they are due to be in theatre for their operation. This is to allow time for the block itself to take effect and time to test whether it covers both the surgical field and the tourniquet site, and for supplementation with more peripheral blocks if this cover is incomplete. The most common reason for failure of nerve plexus blocks is not giving enough time for them to work.

It is usually best to block the large plexuses going to each limb, rather than small peripheral nerves, as it means fewer injections for the patient and often smaller volumes of local anaesthetic being used.

The patient must be able to adopt the correct position to allow the anaesthetist access to the nerve plexus. If a limb is painful to move then splinting it with a blow-up splint can aid positioning. The anaesthetist's assistant can often help in this way by supporting the patient's limb in the correct position either manually or with the help of sandbags or pillows. Holding the limb may help in another way as the assistant may be able to feel muscle fasciculation (twitching) indicating that the anaesthetist's needle has touched the nerve plexus that he is seeking to block.

In the area where the blocks are performed, be it reception area or anaesthetic room, the following equipment should be to hand: local anaesthetic drugs, needles, nerve stimulators, tourniquets, emergency equipment including oxygen and suction equipment and drugs for resuscitation.

Local Anaesthetic Drugs

There should be both short- and long-acting local anaesthetics available. The most usual are bupivacaine, in concentrations of 0.5% (5 mg/ml) and 0.25% (2.5 mg/ml) with and without adrenaline (1:200,000), and lignocaine, in concentrations of 2% (20 mg/ml) and 1% (10 mg/ml) with and without adrenaline (1:200,000).

Prilocaine is the shortest acting (about 2 hours), while lignocaine lasts for about 4 hours and bupivacaine lasts the longest (about 6 hours). Adrenaline can be added for two reasons: to prolong the action of the short-acting compounds (prilocaine and lignocaine) and to reduce the absorption of the drugs into the bloodstream by producing vasoconstriction locally.

The speed of onset varies too. Prilocaine and lignocaine act quickly, within 10–20 min, while bupivacaine may take 30–40 min to produce its full effect.

In practice a mixture of both short-acting and long-acting compounds is often used. This is useful as the short-acting compounds give an early indication that the block is going to work, reassuring to both the patient and the anaesthetist, and the long-acting compound provides prolonged pain freedom in the postoperative period.

For practical purposes the actual dose of the amount of drug used is worked out in the following way:

- Prilocaine: maximum amount = weight (kg) × 6 mg
- Lignocaine: maximum amount = weight (kg) × 4 mg
- Bupivacaine: maximum amount = weight (kg) × 2 mg.

When adrenaline is added to solutions of prilocaine or lignocaine these amounts can be doubled.

For an average-sized male of 70 kg the amounts used correspond therefore to:

- Prilocaine: 420 mg without adrenaline, 840 mg with adrenaline
- Lignocaine: 280 mg without adrenaline, 560 mg with adrenaline
- Bupivacaine: 140 mg with or without adrenaline.

Where a 50:50 mixture is used, half the maximum amount for each drug should not be exceeded. These amounts are designed to prevent excessive absorption into the bloodstream and so prevent toxic reactions.

The toxic reactions of these drugs are on the brain and the heart. In the case of the brain it can lead to convulsions and coma and in the case of the heart to poor cardiac output and circulatory collapse. Treatment must be prompt and may involve circulatory support and general anaesthesia. These are given intra-venously and so the patient must always have an intravenous cannula in place *before the block is done.* If the anaesthetist forgets, do not be afraid to remind him! This precaution should always be adopted because no matter how experienced and careful the anaesthetist is, it might happen that the drug is injected intravenously and this may lead to a toxic response. Because of this ever present danger, blocks should only be performed where resuscitation equipment and facilities for general anaesthesia are immediately to hand. (See Ch. 13).

Needles

Blocks can be done with ordinary hypodermic needles but most anaesthetists prefer to use needles that are less sharp. They give more 'feel' when passing through the sheaths that surround nerve plexuses and, because they are blunter, are less likely to damage nerves or enter blood vessels. These needles, often used as 'spinal' needles, come in various lengths, the most useful begin 5 and 9 cm. Some have markers – sliding plastic discs – which can be positioned to give more accurate placement when using bony landmarks as indicators of depth.

There are specially manufactured 'block' needles, also with a blunt short bevelled tip, which have a length of flexible plastic extension tubing attached. This is so that the weight of the syringe does not make holding the needle in position difficult and allows an easy changeover to a second syringe. An electrical lead is also incorporated in some needles so that a nerve stimulator can be attached. This enables the tip of the needle to impart a stimulus to the nerve plexus it is seeking. When the needle approaches the plexus, twitching is seen in the limb due to the stimulation of motor nerves leading to the muscles. As the sensory nerves run in the same plexus as the motor nerves, injection of local anaesthetic will anaesthetize the limb. The needle tip is at this stage either in the nerve plexus or close enough to allow the local anaesthetic to act upon it. It therefore allows the local anaesthetic to be deposited without the needle actually touching the nerve, a factor some anaesthetists think helps prevent the needle damaging the nerve. When a stimulator is not used, a paraesthesia has to be elicited by actually touching the nerve to be sure the needle is in the right place. It therefore follows that the block must be done on an awake patient so that the patient can inform the anaesthetist when he feels paraesthesia – an electric shock-like feeling. A ground electrode is needed to use one of these needles and an ECG electrode is all that is required for this. It may be that the assistant will be asked to operate the syringe while the anaesthetist holds the needle. The operations will include aspiration (pulling back on the syringe plunger) and injection, and these two actions would only be performed on the instruction of the anaesthetist.

Tourniquet

Both single and double cuff tourniquets should be available, the single for maintaining exsanguination and the double cuff for intravenous regional anaesthesia (Bier's block). Both should be frequently tested to make sure there are no leaks. Deflation of the double cuff is inconvenient as blood is allowed into the wound, but as this double cuff is used for intravenous regional anaesthesia its failure can have dangerous consequences as the local anaesthetic will enter the circulation, and may precipitate toxic consequences for the patient.

Cuffs should be blown up *after* exsanguination *when the arm is in the position that is required for surgery.* If the arm is moved to a wide angle after the cuff is blown up, the nerve plexus which is trapped under the cuff may be stretched and damaged.

In the technique of intravenous anaesthesia (Bier's block) the top cuff (proximal) is blown up first and the lower cuff (distal) blown up 10 min later when the area underneath it is anaesthetized, thus making the presence of the tight cuff much less uncomfortable for the patient.

Tourniquet cuffs are applied over the upper part of the leg or arm simply because they work better there than on the lower half of the limb. This is because there is only one bone here and therefore the blood supply can be effectively abolished. In the lower part of the limb the presence of two bones theoretically prevents compression of the blood supply between them, though in practice a tourniquet works adequately on the lower leg but not so well on the arm. An additional precaution at this site is to make sure the cuff is three finger breadths below the head of the fibula to prevent compression and therefore damage of the peroneal nerve. Exsanguination of the limb prior to applying the tourniquet is achieved by wrapping an elasticized rubber bandage (Esmarch) tightly round the limb up to the level of the tourniquet and unwinding the bandage or by use of a rubber exsanguinator device.

Cuff pressure and duration

Theoretically the cuff should be 50 mmHg above the patients systolic blood pressure. In adults, this means a pressure of around 200 mmHg in the arm and 300 mmHg in the leg. The times that the cuff is blown up for should not exceed 2 hours for the arm and 3 hours for the leg. Times should be accurately recorded for when the cuff is blown up and released.

Miscellaneous equipment

Sandbags, foam wedges and pillows should be available to help position the patient and make maintenance of that position as comfortable as possible. A seat or stool should be available for the anaesthetist so that the anaesthetist, by being comfortable himself, is able to hold the needle as steadily as possible when performing the block. Jet-splints are useful in casualty/emergency theatres where blocks may have to be performed on fractured and therefore painful limbs. These splints make painful limbs more easy to position. A personal stereo helps distract the patient from the extraneous noises in the theatre and helps the patient to relax. This is a cheap reusable anaesthetic aid and should not be thought of as a luxury. If the patient is awake it is important to have a method of screening the operation from the patient's view. This can usually be provided by the attachment of a right-angled bar to the theatre table, and positioning a theatre drape over it.

Commonest Blocks

The most frequently used major nerve blocks in regional anaesthesia for surgery are:

- Brachial plexus block – interscalene; supracalvicular and axillary approaches
- Sciatic nerve block – posterior, anterior and popliteal approaches
- Femoral nerve block – either alone, or as part of a 3-in-1 block
- Lumbosacral plexus block – psoas or fascia iliaca compartment block.

Minor nerve blocks frequently employed for pain relief are intercostal nerve blocks for thoracic and abdominal surgery; ilio-inguinal/ilio-hypogastric nerve blocks for hernia operations; lateral cutaneous nerve blocks for split skin grafts from the high: penile nerve blocks for circumcision. Blocks for the nerves at the ankle and wrist (sural, superficial peroneal, posterior tibial, ulnar, median, radial) are often used to cover operations on the fingers and toes. Blocks at the elbow and knee are not so commonly used although they can be very useful as supplements to more proximal plexus blocks.

When nerve blocks are the sole anaesthetic it is important to remember that not all sensation may be removed. While pain sensation may have disappeared, deep touch and vibration may be felt or transmitted and the patient should be informed of this either prior to the block or at the time of it being applied. It is not helpful to keep asking the patient if he/she can feel anything. Allow the anaesthetist to judge this from the patient's response to tourniquet, testing (by pinching) or surgery. If the block is not absolutely perfect, the administration of intravenous analgesics and/or sedatives plus a small amount of local anaesthetic infiltration by the surgeon can leave the patient untroubled by the surgery. Nitrous oxide inhalation can also be very helpful in providing supplementary analgesia and sedation.

Postoperatively instructions must be written by the anaesthetist to the effect that the limb must be protected for at least four hours after the block has been put in place. The patient cannot feel or move the limb and so it must be protected from lying against hard surfaces and prevented from hanging over the edge of the trolley or bed.

SEDATION TECHNIQUES IN REGIONAL ANAESTHESIA

T. D. McCubbin

The choice of sedation for a regional technique is of great importance if the full benefit of the local nerve block is to be realized. The aim of any sedation technique in this context is to decrease anxiety, and to produce a relaxed but cooperative patient whilst the nerve block is being performed and the surgical procedure carried out. In different circumstances the amount of sedation required will vary from none at all to a full general anaesthetic. Every patient presenting for operation under a regional technique has to be carefully assessed preoperatively by the anaesthetist who should be prepared to change from one form of sedation to another if the need arises. The need for, and the most appropriate type of, sedation will generally depend upon the patient, the type of operation being performed and the individual anaesthetist concerned.

The Patient

Preference

It is particularly important in regional anaesthetic techniques to explain fully to the patient preoperatively details of the nerve block that is to be performed and of how this will prevent any feeling of discomfort during the surgical procedure. Patients may initially demonstrate a reluctance to be awake during a surgical operation. In such cases it is important to reassure the patient that sedation will be available as required to completely allay their anxiety whilst in the operating theatre. The type of surgery may influence the motivation of the patient to remain fully conscious, as in a Caesarean section for example. The anaesthetist must always be available during the procedure to modify the degree of sedation if required. In this context it is extremely helpful if the anaesthetic assistant remains with the patient during the operation and can if required, and the patient desires, chat to them during the surgery.

Associated medical conditions

If the patient is suffering from other medical conditions, this may indicate the need for more or less sedation. Patients suffering from unrelated orthopaedic conditions may find prolonged immobility on the operating table unpleasant, with a requirement for more sedation. On the other hand, in patients suffering from chronic respiratory disease, it may be prudent to limit the amount of sedation given.

Age

Young children may require a general anaesthetic to cover a regional technique whilst elderly patients tend to be more stoical.

Degree of anxiety

In patients who remain extremely nervous even after a proper explanation of the procedure, it may occasionally be necessary to resort to a general anaesthetic.

The Operation

The first consideration must be – is the operation suitable for a regional technique under sedation? Epidural blocks are used in some centres for major aortic surgery. Such cases require controlled ventilation during surgery and the block therefore has to be covered by a full general anaesthetic.

Consideration must be given as to whether the performance of the nerve block itself may require sedation. This could arise for example in a patient with a fractured neck of femur having a spinal anaesthetic where turning into the required position may be very painful.

The duration of the operation has to be taken into account. The longer the procedure, the greater is likely to be the need for sedation, as will be the case where the patient is positioned in lithotomy for example.

With the increasing use of day case surgery, a quick recovery is obviously desirable. This may indicate the need to limit the sedation and to use short-acting drugs.

The success rate of any particular nerve block has to be taken into account. In general terms, spinal blocks tend to be highly effective and the need for sedation may be reduced. Upper and lower limb blocks may not be as effective and may take considerably longer to develop. In this latter case more sedation may be required.

Technique of Sedation

Commonly used drugs

For sedating awake patients the drugs available may be divided into pure sedatives, which usually have no analgesic properties, and opioids, which are primarily analgesics but have sedative effects as well.

Benzodiazepines are the most commonly used. They may be given orally, intramuscularly or intravenously. The intravenous route allows the degree of sedation to be titrated against the patients response. These drugs have certain disadvantages. They tend to be long acting, and they have potent amnesic properties which may be an advantage, but which may also be undesirable in the case of a Caesarean section. They tend to be unsatisfactory for sedating patients who are in pain or discomfort.

Opioids are the drugs of choice if the patient complains of pain or discomfort. Again, the intravenous route of administration allows a more rapid response particularly with the shorter-acting agents such as fentanyl or alfentanil. These compounds should be used in combination with an anti-emetic to prevent nausea or vomiting during surgery.

Infusions of intravenous anaesthetics such as propofol can also be used to provide varying degrees of sedation but again without any analgesia. The infusion of intravenous anaesthetic may also produce over-sedation, with consequent difficulties in airway control.

Recently, patient-controlled sedation with benzodiazepines or propofol has been described.

If a decision is made to use general anaesthesia to cover a regional technique, then the level of anaesthesia should be sufficient to keep the patient asleep whilst maintaining spontaneous ventilation unless controlled ventilation is indicated. Tracheal intubation is usually unnecessary and the airway can be maintained either with a mask and/or an oral airway or a laryngeal mask airway. In most cases it is probably preferable and safer to perform the regional block before inducing general anaesthesia. The use of taped music with patient earphones may provide good relaxation with a reduction in the need for sedative drugs.

Inhalational sedation and analgesia with nitrous oxide can be very helpful.

Problems – Intraoperative

Unfortunately the conscious state may prove disadvantageous in the patient undergoing surgery in cases where the patient is hostile and uncooperative. Such patients may move around during the procedure or even attempt to leave the operating table. In these circumstances the patient is likely to receive increasing amounts of sedative and hypnotic drugs until a state of general anaesthesia is produced with none of the benefits of a formal and planned general anaesthetic technique. However, this situation should rarely arise if the points made above are fully considered.

It is important for all theatre staff to remember that the patient is awake, and therefore general conversation and remarks should be guarded. The contribution of the anaesthetic assistant in the management of these cases should not be underestimated. The assistant can do much to reinforce the preoperative reassurance which the anaesthetist has provided. Intraoperatively the presence of an understanding assistant who can explain precisely what is happening to the patient is of immense value in allaying anxiety and making the patient feel more comfortable. Postoperatively it is important for the anaesthetist to visit the patient and ensure complete satisfaction.

In most cases the patient will be more than happy to have a future surgical operation carried out under a regional technique if this seems appropriate.

KEY LEARNING POINTS

1. The anaesthetist's assistant has a vital role to play in helping with the safe and correct conduct of local and regional anaesthesia.

2. Discuss with the anaesthetist what will be needed in terms of equipment, drugs, monitoring and patient positioning.

3. Ensure that you are always prepared to assist with the treatment of local anaesthetic toxicity and a 'total spinal block'.

4. Be prepared for intervention to convert to a general anaesthetic technique.

5. In children, local and regional anaesthesia is now widely used and the same principles apply.

Further Reading

'Principles and practice of regional anaesthesia', 2nd edition. Edited by JAW Wildsmith, EN Armitage. Churchill Livingstone, Edinburgh, 1993.

Relevance

ODP Level 3   Units 3, 4, 5, 6, 8.

SECTION 3

MAINTENANCE AND MONITORING

5. MAINTENANCE AND MONITORING OF THE AIRWAY AND THE ADEQUACY OF VENTILATION

N. S. Morton

During maintenance of anaesthesia, keeping the airway open is critical to ensure adequate delivery of oxygen and anaesthetic gases and adequate carbon dioxide removal. If the airway is not open, the oxygen supply to the patient's lungs will be impaired and transfer of oxygen to arterial blood and to the body tissues will decrease. Within minutes the lack of oxygen supply to brain, heart, muscle and other vital organs will cause damage. At the same time, CO_2 elimination from the lungs will be impeded and the CO_2 concentration in the blood will build up. High CO_2 concentrations stimulate the breathing centre in the brain and cause an increase in heart rate, irritability of the heart muscle, an increase in blood pressure and increased blood flow to the brain. Very high concentrations of CO_2 in the blood cause coma and eventually depression of breathing.

Airway obstruction also results in a decrease in the delivery of anaesthetic gases (nitrous oxide and volatile agents) to the lungs, blood and brain and the depth of anaesthesia thus tends to lighten. This can lead to serious problems such as awareness, consciousness, movement, coughing or laryngeal spasm.

Thus maintenance of a patent airway is a fundamental principle of patient safety during anaesthesia. The anaesthetist must match his technique for maintaining the airway to the individual patient, taking into account age, medical problems, surgical procedure and requirements, and the duration and type of anaesthesia.

In the spontaneous breathing patient, five main options are available. The simplest is where the patient maintains their own airway when undergoing a procedure under local or regional anaesthetic, either with no sedation or light sedation, administered intravenously by the anaesthetist (e.g. small bolus doses or a low dose infusion of midazolam or propofol) or by patient-controlled infusion. Light inhalational sedation with nitrous oxide in oxygen for pain relief in labour or for dental sedation is another example where the aim is to have the patient maintaining their own airway.

How do you decide in such a case whether the airway is adequate? Clinical signs are the best, but electronic monitors are helpful. The basic symptoms and signs to check are:

- is the patient making breathing movements?
- are these breathing movements at a normal rate for this patient?
- are the breathing movements of a normal pattern?
- is breathing noisy or wheezy?
- is the colour of the patient's lips and tongue pink or not?

Obviously if the patient is not making breathing movements, this is an emergency which needs to be rectified by basic and advanced life support. Cessation of breathing may be due to an overdose of sedatives or a complication of the local or regional anaesthesia.

If breathing movements are present, the rate of breathing is a helpful clinical sign but must be interpreted for different age groups, for example small children normally have a fast breathing rate. Very rapid, shallow breathing is not normal and very slow breathing rates usually indicate oversedation, particularly when opioid drugs have been given.

The pattern of breathing is very helpful: the chest and abdomen should rise and fall together. If they do not, it usually implies that the airway is partly or completely obstructed and a 'see-saw' pattern of movement of the chest and abdomen is seen (Fig. 5.1).

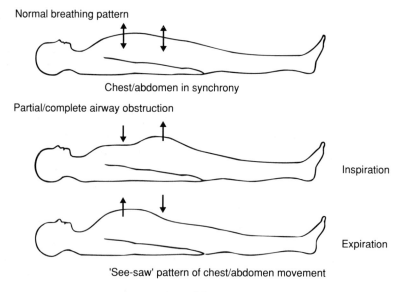

Fig. 5.1 'See-saw' pattern of chest and abdomen movements

This is because the diaphragm contracts and moves down pushing the contents of the abdomen down and out. With the airway obstructed gas cannot be drawn down the airway easily to fill the lungs and expand the chest, so the chest does not rise. If airway obstruction is severe, the chest wall may even be pulled inwards because the diaphragm muscle is attached to the inner surface of the lower ribs. The 'see-saw' breathing pattern is a very sinister sign and efforts must be taken at once to open the airway.

Noisy breathing (stridor) usually indicates a partly obstructed airway and is often accompanied by a 'see-saw' breathing pattern. Stridor during inspiration usually means upper airway obstruction while stridor or wheeze during expiration usually means lower airway obstruction in the trachea or large bronchi or narrowing of small airways, for example in asthma.

Cyanosis or blueness of the tongue or lips indicates low oxygen levels in the blood. This is a late sign and there needs to be at least 5 g of deoxygenated haemoglobin per 100 ml of blood to become obvious. If the patient is very anaemic this clinical sign will appear even later. Cyanosis, along with some of the other signs noted above, indicates critical airway obstruction.

So clinical signs in the spontaneously breathing unintubated patient give the quickest/earliest clues to airway obstruction. Electronic monitoring is helpful but changes in monitored values such as oxygen saturation, heart rate and ECG tend to occur later, once airway obstruction has been present for some time.

In the anaesthetized spontaneously breathing patient, the airway can be maintained by facemask and jaw support with the addition of an oral airway if needed. Another option is to use the laryngeal mask airway (LMA). As well as clinical signs and pulse oximetry, the use of an anaesthetic circuit with a reservoir bag adds further possibilities for monitoring. The movement of the reservoir bag in time with breathing movements is a helpful visual clue. A gas analyser can be included in the circuit, which allows measurement of the inspired and expired gas concentrations flows and volumes. This allows more accurate assessment of the patency of the airway and the adequacy of ventilation. In particular the graph of the carbon dioxide breathed in and out (the capnograph) gives much useful information. If the lungs are normal, and assuming no leaks in the circuit, the peak level of expired CO_2 (end tidal CO_2) gives an indication of the adequacy of ventilation.

The airway can also be secured by tracheal intubation and all the above monitoring techniques can be used. Where ventilation is controlled, electronic monitoring becomes more important as many of the clinical signs are lost. The symmetry of chest movement and movement in time with the ventilator cycles is useful. An increase in the peak airway pressure can indicate airway obstruction, for example blocked/kinked tracheal tube. The capnograph waveform confirms the integrity and patency of the artificial airway and the adequacy of ventilation. Most ventilators and monitors allow measurement and display of the volume of each breath in and out, its gas composition, the rate of ventilation and calculate the volume of expired gas per minute.

Another simple clinical monitor of ventilation is to listen to the breath sounds with a stethoscope and in the intubated patient listening to each side of the chest to check for equality confirms that the tracheal tube is correctly positioned in the trachea and there is no pneumothorax or lung collapse.

6. MAINTENANCE AND MONITORING OF THE CIRCULATION

H. Hosie, N. S. Morton

WHAT IS 'THE CIRCULATION' AND WHY DO WE NEED IT?

The evolution of complex organisms made up of lots of cells from single-celled creatures in prehistoric times has depended on the evolution of a system for delivery of nutrients to and removal of toxic wastes from every cell of the organism. In humans, like many other creatures, the transport medium is blood and the network system is the circulation.

The Transport Medium

Blood is made up of cellular particles suspended in a liquid – the plasma. The plasma is a protein-rich solution which also contains salt ions and essential nutrients. These are glucose and other simple sugars, amino acids, fatty acids, trace elements and minerals which are needed to maintain cell function. It also contains products of metabolism, such as urea and carbon dioxide. These are carried to specialized organs, such as the lungs or kidneys and liver, which remove toxic waste products from the body.

The cells in the blood are: red cells (erythrocytes), which carry oxygen molecules; white cells (leukocytes), which are involved in defence reactions against foreign particles or cells; and platelets, which are involved in clot formation. The red cells contain the pigment haemoglobin, which carries oxygen from the lungs to the tissues.

The Network System

The anatomy of the circulation at first appears complex but can be thought of as two separate systems which exchange contents at the pumping station (the heart). A pump is necessary to push the transport medium around the network (Fig. 6.1).

The systemic circulation distributes oxygen-rich blood to every cell in the body from the left ventricle of the heart, through the aorta and the major

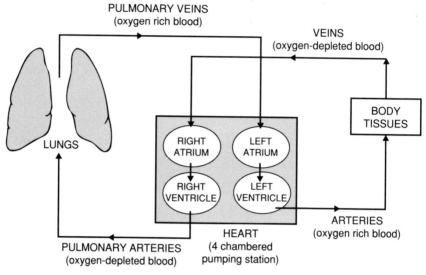

Fig. 6.1 *The circulation*

arteries to the smaller arterioles and finally to the tiny capillaries which lie very close to the cells of every tissue in the body. The cells take up oxygen and other nutrients from the arterial blood and pass carbon dioxide and other products of metabolism to the blood lying in the capillaries. This oxygen-depleted blood containing waste products is moved on around the circulation from the capillaries to small venules and larger and larger veins to drain through the inferior or superior vena cava into the right side of the heart.

During your work in theatre you will have plenty of opportunity to see the differences between arterial and venous blood, either at formal cannulation or during surgery. Arterial blood is usually bright red, indicating it is carrying lots of oxygen, it spurts from the artery under high pressure and can fill a syringe without the need for aspiration. Arterial puncture is performed by palpation of the artery and insertion of the needle. Venous blood is a much darker colour, indicating that it has given up the oxygen stores, it oozes from a wound and has to be aspirated from a peripheral vein. To perform venepuncture the flow of blood through the vein is blocked and the vein proximal to the obstruction fills with blood. This allows the vein to be palpated and punctured by the needle.

The oxygen-depleted blood which has returned to the right side of the heart needs to pick up fresh supplies of oxygen from the lungs. It is pumped by the right ventricle through the lungs, through the pulmonary artery and arterioles to capillaries lying in close contact with the air-filled alveoli of the lungs. As blood passes through these capillaries, oxygen moves from the air-filled spaces across the alveolar membrane into the capillary and binds with the haemoglobin molecules in the red blood cells. At the same time the carbon dioxide waste passes out of the capillaries into the alveoli and will be breathed out on expiration. The oxygenated blood then travels through the pulmonary venules to the pulmonary veins before emptying into the left side of the heart. The left ventricle then pumps the oxygenated blood back into the systemic circulation to provide the cells with further supplies of oxygen.

The primary function of the circulation in man is to supply oxygen to the tissues of the body. Some tissues can continue to function for a period of time, but without oxygen the cells ultimately die. This is what happens in peripheral vascular disease where lack of oxygen supply due to narrowed and inadequate blood vessels result in areas of tissue necrosis or gangrene. The organ which is most sensitive to oxygen lack is the brain whose cells can only survive a few minutes without oxygen before dying. As brain cells cannot repair themselves, this damage is permanent and ultimately leads to hypoxic brain damage, persistent vegetative state or death. A number of mechanisms exist to protect the brain, the heart and the kidneys, which are also known as the 'vital organs', and these are described below.

Maintenance of Circulation

From the description above, it is clear that the supply of oxygen to the various tissues is vital. However, the oxygen demands of the various tissues are not constant but variable. For instance the oxygen demand from your leg muscles when you are sitting still is less than that needed when walking. More oxygen still is needed when vigorous exercise is being carried out. The circulation has to be able to provide more oxygen to areas of need and consequently divert blood from one area to another, depending on the body activity.

The key to understanding the circulation is understanding the changes in blood flow in the body. The flow of blood to any area of the body is, like the flow of any liquid in a tube, dependent upon the pressure pushing the liquid round and the diameter of the tube. Flow is less through a narrow tube than through a wide tube. In the body the blood vessels can dilate (grow larger) or constrict (narrow) as a result of activity of the autonomic nervous system. This nervous system supplies nerves to the arterioles and veins of the circulation. Constriction of the arterioles increases the resistance to flow (increased systemic vascular resistance or SVR) and so reduces blood flow to that area. Constriction of the veins empties blood out of that area (decreased capacitance) and back into the circulation. The pressure driving the blood round the circulation is dependent upon the activity of the heart, which is also supplied by nerves from the autonomic nervous system. The heart can vary how fast it pumps (the heart rate) and how much blood it pumps at each beat (the stroke volume). Within certain limits as the heart beats faster, the blood flow will increase and as the heart empties more completely with each beat the blood flow will further increase.

The heart, brain and kidneys are vital organs and their oxygen supply must be protected to keep the body functioning. These organs 'autoregulate'. This means that over a range of blood pressure normally found in an individual the blood vessel size varies to keep the blood flow constant and it is only when the pressure becomes very low or very high that there is any change in blood flow to these organs.

This description of the anatomy and physiology of the circulation is very brief and the subject is complex. Anaesthesia and disease can affect the normal control mechanisms and surgery induces change in the circulation.

Monitoring the Circulation

Monitoring the circulation under anaesthesia is vital to the anaesthetist because of potential changes due to anaesthesia, surgery, and disease. The techniques in common use are outlined below.

Because oxygen is carried mainly by the red blood cells and is dependent on both the number of red cells and their haemoglobin content, assessment of the blood is made by counting the number of red cells (red cell count) and measuring the haemoglobin content of the blood. Normal levels depend upon age, sex, smoking habits and disease processes, but most anaesthetists would wish haemoglobin levels of 100 g/l (10 g/dl) or greater and would transfuse to maintain this level. There are exceptions to this rule such as in patients with chronic kidney failure. Full blood counts are performed by the haematology laboratories but approximations can be made using arterial blood gas machines, co-oximeters or from spinning a capillary sample to give the packed cell volume (PCV). Because of protective physiological mechanisms, full blood counts done during major haemorrhage may not be accurate and may need to be repeated.

Blood volume can be assessed by calculating total blood volume for the patient (about 70 ml/kg in an adult) and measuring the blood losses. This is particularly important in children whose blood volume is very small and even tiny blood losses can be significant. Weighing of swabs and measuring suction losses is vital in assessing blood loss and the anaesthetist should be alerted if blood losses are being lost into drapes, gowns or the floor as these losses are often not recorded formally. Blood volume can be assessed by measuring the changes in central venous pressure although this has limitations.

The heart action is assessed by using the electrocardiograph to assess heart rate and rhythm, measuring the arterial pressure to ensure an adequate pumping pressure or more invasively using pulmonary artery flotation catheters to measure cardiac output and stroke volume. More simply, information on the pump action can be obtained by palpating a peripheral artery and noting the frequency and strength of the pulse.

Blood flow can be simply assessed by the colour of the patient and particularly by examination of the extremities such as the finger tips or toes. If blood flow is good they will be warm and pink. The capillary refill time is a useful measure. The finger or toe is squeezed until it blanches and the rate of return of pink colour gives an estimate of peripheral blood flow. Anaesthesia has been revolutionized by the development of pulse oximetry which gives information on both blood flow and oxygenation.

Monitoring the Blood Volume

Central venous pressure (CVP)

The central venous pressure is the pressure of blood measured at the junction of the vena cava with the right atrium. The pressure fluctuates with breathing as it reflects pressure inside the chest and it also varies with the contraction of the right atrium and movement of the tricuspid valve. It is also dependent upon hydrostatic forces and is affected by the position of the patient. In addition to being used as a measure of blood volume it also reflects right ventricular function.

Central venous lines are inserted if large blood losses have occurred or are anticipated so that rapid infusion of blood or fluid may be given and an assessment of needs for further transfusion made. Central lines are also used for the delivery of hypertonic fluids or drugs and may be inserted in procedures where air embolism is possible (e.g. neurosurgery in the head-up position).

Central venous lines are inserted via either the right or left internal jugular vein or the right or left subclavian veins. Occasionally they may be inserted via the femoral veins. The cannula is usually advanced so that the tip lies at the junction of the vena cava with the right atrium although for treatment of air embolus it is pushed in further. Anaesthetists will have a preference for sites of puncture but it is more usual for the right internal jugular vein to be used when the patient is to have a general anaesthetic and controlled ventilation because of the lower risk of pneumothorax using this approach. Exceptions are in neurosurgery or head and neck surgery where an arm vein or leg vein would be preferred.

Preparation of the patient

Central venous lines may be inserted using an aseptic technique under local anaesthesia or after induction of general anaesthesia. The patient must be tipped head down, as air may be drawn into the circulation if the central venous pressure is low, causing an air embolism. The patient's head is then turned away from the side of entry for the jugular approach and this demonstrates the sternocleidomastoid muscle which can be used as a landmark. The skin is prepared and cleaned and the area draped. Methods vary between anaesthetists but there is a trend towards using the Seldinger technique to insert the line. This uses a 'seeking' needle to identify the vessel, through which passes a guide wire. The guide wire is flexible at one end and should not puncture the vessel wall. Once the guide wire is passed, the seeking needle is withdrawn. If the cannula is large, such as a triple lumen catheter, an incision may need to be made in the skin and a dilator used to dilate up the puncture site to enable the catheter to pass into the vessel. The catheter is then passed over the stiff end of the guide wire into the vessel and the guide wire removed. The catheter is then fixed in place.

Complications

Complications that may arise are:

- air drawn into the vein (air embolism)
- artery puncture
- pneumothorax
- arrhythmias
- perforation of the vein or heart
- haemothorax
- haematoma in the neck
- chylothorax (due to damage to the thoracic duct which carries lymphatic fluid (chyle) from the tissues to the veins).

Interpretation

Normal CVP values range between 0 and 10 mmHg when the transducer is zeroed at the right atrium. Low CVP suggests reduced blood volume or vasodilatation. High CVP suggests fluid overload, vasoconstriction or right heart failure. CVP is also raised as a result of artificial ventilation, coughing or if air, blood or fluid is present in the thorax or mediastinum.

Monitoring Pump Function

Pulse

Despite using increasingly sophisticated monitors, palpating the pulse is a simple and effective way of assessing the adequacy of the circulation. A palpable pulse confirms an adequate blood flow when automatic monitoring devices give error messages or malfunction. Pulse points are felt wherever an artery lies near the surface and can be compressed against a bone. Typical sites are the radial artery at the wrist on the thumb side of the hand, the brachial artery at the elbow, the facial or temporal arteries in the head, the carotid artery in the neck, dorsalis pedis or the posterior tibial artery in the foot and the femoral artery in the groin. Check you know where all these pulse points are (Fig. 6.2).

The pulse gives information about the rhythm, which can be regular or irregular, and the heart rate, which can be normal, fast or slow. It may also give some information about the arterial pressure. If the pulse is strong the

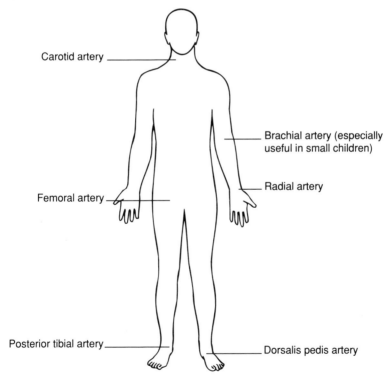

Fig. 6.2 Pulse points

pressure will be normal or high; if the pulse is difficult to feel, weak or thready, the pressure is likely to be low. If electronic monitors display abnormalities or alarm, train yourself to look first at the patient, check their colour and feel for a pulse whilst checking for other causes.

Listening with a stethoscope

As well as being useful in confirming breath sounds, the stethoscope can give valuable information about the heart. Listening to the heart sounds confirms the rhythm and also gives information about abnormal sounds such as the 'mill wheel' murmur occasionally heard when air embolism occurs. Stethoscopes can be sited over the chest wall (precordially) or in the oesophagus. they are most often used in paediatric practice.

Electrocardiograph (ECG)

The ECG or electrocardiograph monitors electrical activity arising from contraction and relaxation of heart muscle. ECGs are part of the minimal monitoring needed for every patient having anaesthesia.

What is an ECG?

All muscles contract as a result of movement of ions across cell membranes. Movements of ions gives rise to tiny electrical discharges. These can be detected by electrodes on the body surface, the signals amplified and characteristic waveforms produced. An ECG is a series of waves relating to activity within the heart. Most heartbeats give rise to a P wave, a QRS complex and a T wave. The P wave corresponds to the electrical activity from contraction of the right and left atria. The QRS complex is the electrical activity from contraction of the right and left ventricles and the repolarization of the atria. The T wave corresponds to the repolarization of the ventricles.

The PQRST complex may look different in different patients as the size and shape of the complexes depend on the location of the detector electrodes in relation to the heart. A conventional 12-lead ECG tracing produces 12 different 'views' of the heart using 12 standard combinations from detectors on the right and left arms and the left leg and six chest leads located at standard positions round the chest wall. Information obtained from a 12-lead ECG includes rhythm, previous ischaemia or infarcts, conduction disturbances, electrolyte disturbances and hypertrophy or strain of the chambers of the heart. It is, however, a snapshot of the cardiac activity and a normal ECG does not necessarily mean that the heart is healthy.

More commonly in theatre and recovery a continuous ECG is used to monitor cardiac function. Most cardiac monitors are able to monitor leads I,

II, aVr, aV1, aVf and a chest lead dependent on the siting of the electrodes. It is often recommended that lead II be selected routinely as this lead is used for interpreting rhythm disturbances. In patients at high risk of heart attack it is recommended that a CMV5 lead is used. One electrode should be placed at the manubrium (breastbone), one at the V5 position on the chest (the fifth interspace on the anterior axillary line) and the other on the left shoulder.

Preparation of patient

With modern pregelled electrodes skin preparation is less important than in the past. Certain patients may need patches of hair removed for humanitarian reasons (it will be sore removing the electrodes) and to get good contact with the skin. Poor quality ECGs may also be the result of dry electrodes. From the explanation above it will be clear that the positioning of the electrodes in some patients will be of importance. This is particularly true in cardiac surgery and ECG technicians may set up the ECG in these cases. It may be useful to tape over the electrodes to stop blood or skin preparation fluids from getting under the electrode, especially if the site of surgery is near the electrodes.

Interpretation

It is outside the scope of this book to describe in detail abnormalities which may be seen on the continuous ECG, and interpretation can be difficult. However, it can show extra abnormal beats, abnormal rhythms, which may be fast or slow, regular or irregular, and changes in the ST segment, which may indicate possible ischaemia (oxygen deprivation). It is important to realize that continuing electrical activity of the heart does not mean that the heart is pumping blood effectively. For example, in the condition of electro-mechanical dissociation (EMD), the heart continues to generate electrical impulses but no pumping action is occurring and the patient has no pulse to feel.

Pulmonary artery flotation catheter (PAFC)

Pulmonary artery flotation catheters are also known as Swan Ganz catheters. They have a balloon at their tip which enables the catheter to be 'floated' through the right ventricle to lie in the pulmonary artery. The tip lies in a small arteriole and when the balloon is inflated it stops the blood flow temporarily. The pressure at the tip of the catheter then reflects the pressure in the left atrium of the heart and is known as the pulmonary capillary wedge pressure (PCWP).

In addition to measuring the PCWP, insertion of a PAFC can allow cardiac output measurements to be calculated, which can be useful in patients in shock or with severely diseased hearts.

Preparation of the patient

PFACs are inserted in a similar manner to central venous lines and the same preparations apply. However, these catheters are often of a wider bore than central lines and are inserted through a large bore introducer with a protective sterile sheath to maintain sterility of the catheter. Positioning of the catheter correctly depends upon interpreting a transduced pressure tracing on a monitor and the appropriate transducers must be available. Measurement of cardiac output requires either a special injection system or a special continuous-reading catheter. This technique is highly sophisticated and is used in specific, specialized situations such as the patient with severe heart disease or the patient with shock.

Monitoring the Blood Flow

Pulse oximeter

The pulse oximeter confirms the presence of a pulse (and hence a cardiac output) and the degree of saturation of the blood. It is a sensitive beat to beat monitor of cardiac output, blood flow and oxygenation. It is now considered an essential piece of monitoring for anaesthesia, sedation and recovery.

Sites for monitoring

Any finger or toe can be used with a finger probe. Care must be taken to ensure that outside light cannot hit the probe as that gives rise to a poor quality signal. Special disposable adhesive neonatal finger and toe probes are available. Other probes have been developed for attachment to earlobes or adhesive disposable probes for the bridge of the nose. In babies and in patients having long-term monitoring using the pulse oximeter, skin damage and burning have been reported and so periodic checks should be made of the probe site.

Interpretation

Arterial oxygen saturation should be more than 90%. Venous blood is usually 75% saturated. Action should be taken if the arterial oxygen saturation suddenly drops or if it is persistently low. Pulse oximeters frequently alarm if there are rapid changes in arterial pressure or if there is hypotension (low blood pressure). If there are problems with obtaining a reading check the BP. Patient movement and shivering also may interfere with the reading and, rarely the patient with abnormal haemoglobin will give false results. Certain dyes (e.g. methylene blue) also give false readings and even nail varnish can cause problems.

Blood pressure

The 'blood pressure' is more correctly the arterial pressure as it is the pressure generated by contraction of the left ventricle of the heart and transmitted along the arteries. It is measured in a peripheral artery, usually in a limb, and may be indirect (non-invasive) or direct (invasive) via a cannula inserted directly into an artery.

The easiest way to monitor the arterial pressure is to palpate an artery at a pulse point as described earlier. If the automatic sphygmomanometer alarms during surgery or in recovery always try to feel a peripheral pulse whilst checking the reading. If it is difficult to feel and the machine is giving low readings it is likely that the drop in pressure is important.

When a peripheral artery is palpated intermittent pulses of pressure are felt. This corresponds to the beat of the heart. In between beats, blood is still flowing in the artery but as the pressure is less it is impossible to feel. When you measure the arterial pressure you measure the maximum pressure (at the beat) and the pressure between beats. The pressure generated when the ventricle of the heart is contracting is the systolic pressure, while the ventricular relaxation is known as diastole. Thus recordings of arterial pressure usually have two numbers, the higher is the systolic pressure and the lower the diastolic pressure.

Anaesthetists may also talk about the mean pressure. Mean usually means average but because more time is spent in diastole than systole the mean arterial pressure is not the arithmetical average of the two numbers. It is often calculated by automatic sphygmomanometers or displayed in direct arterial line measurements. It is used as a measure of blood supply to the vital organs.

Arterial pressures in children are low, with systolic pressures of 80–100 mmHg common in babies and a gradual increase throughout childhood. By adulthood systolic pressures are usually within the range of 100–150 mmHg. Further increases are seen with age and the elderly have higher pressures still and are less able to tolerate hypotension (low arterial pressure).

Indirect or non-invasive methods

These methods all use the principle that obstructed flow is turbulent and therefore noisy, whereas blood flow in arteries is usually smooth and laminar and therefore quiet.

To understand the difference between turbulent and laminar flow, think of a garden hose with the water turned on. If you stand on the hose it is obstructed. As you lift your foot off the hose, water begins to flow and makes a noise because initially the flow is turbulent. Once you lift off your foot completely the obstruction to flow is released and normal water flow resumes. This is known as laminar or smooth flow and is quiet.

Non-invasive measurement of arterial pressure uses a sphygmomanometer cut wrapped round a limb to obstruct blood flow in the arteries of that limb. A variety of detectors can be used to sense the beginning of turbulent flow, which corresponds to systolic pressure, and to detect the change to laminar flow, which corresponds to diastolic pressure. At its simplest, indirect measurement of pressure uses a sphygmomanometer cuff and a stethoscope. The cuff is applied to a limb and inflated above systolic pressure, that is until you cannot palpate the peripheral artery distal to the cuff. The stethoscope is laid over an artery and the pressure slowly reduced. As the pressure reaches systolic values, some blood will leak past the cuff at systole.

Because the flow is turbulent it is noisy and can be heard with the stethoscope. It sounds like a knocking noise. That pressure is noted and recorded as the systolic pressure. As the pressure falls further more blood leaks past the cuff and the quality of the noise changes. It generally grows louder and then becomes more muffled before disappearing altogether. The pressure when the sounds become muffled is usually recorded as the diastolic pressure.

Automatic sphygmomanometers use the same principle of an inflatable cuff but use a variety of detectors, including second cuffs or microphones. Appropriate cuffs must be used for the patient ranging from the tiny neonatal cuffs to extra-large cuffs for an adult thigh. If the cuff does not encircle the limb completely the pressure will not be even and inaccurate recordings will be made. Alarms and settings on automatic sphygmomanometers must be set for the particular patient. Different settings are needed for neonates and alarms must be checked to be appropriate for each patient.

Direct or invasive methods

This technique uses a cannula inserted into a peripheral artery to transmit the arterial pressure waveform via a fluid-filled line to a transducer. Movements within the transducer are interpreted electronically to give a waveform displayed on a monitor screen (see Fig. 2.8). The pressures generated are compared to an internal calibration and are also displayed on screen. This will give a beat to beat measurement of the arterial pressure and is particularly useful in critically ill patients or in procedures where sudden changes in pressure are sometimes seen (see Ch. 2).

Sites for insertion

The most commonly used artery is the radial artery of the non-dominant hand, but other sites include the brachial artery, dorsalis pedis artery, posterior tibial artery and the femoral artery. Problems can arise with arterial cannulation, particularly if the artery is small. The blood supply distal to the artery can be impaired and careful supervision of the line is essential. Allen's test may be performed before cannulating the radial artery, in order to check the adequacy of the ulnar artery supply to the hand. This is done by occluding both vessels by pressing on them and releasing the ulnar pressure. If the hand pinks up quickly the ulnar artery supply is probably adequate. The non-dominant hand is preferred so that less functional damage would be inflicted if the blood flow to the hand was impaired.

Preparation of the patient

Arterial cannulation can be done under local anaesthesia prior to induction of general anaesthesia or once the patient has gone to sleep. Anaesthetists have their own preferences depending on the patient and type of operation. Adult cannulae are 20G or less, paediatric cannulae 22 or 24G. Some cannulae come with a guide wire and use a Seldinger technique, while more conventional methods rely upon puncturing the artery and threading the cannula along it. Heparinized saline is needed to flush the cannula to prevent clots forming and the cannula is fixed in position either with secure strapping or using a stitch before being connected to a heparinized saline-filled manometer line. These lines are connected to flush devices which continuously flush tiny amounts of heparinized saline through the line to maintain its patency. The line is connected to a transducer which is fluid filled and conducts pressure waves from the artery to a flexible diaphragm. The movements of the diaphragm are converted to an electrical signal and displayed upon the monitor. Transducers can be reusable or disposable. Any bubbles of air in the line or transducer will be compressed by the pulsation pressure and so reduce the pressure transmitted to the diaphragm. This leads to a flattened trace and is known as damping. Transducers and monitoring lines have many connections and at least one three-way tap for blood sampling. It is imperative to check the security of all connections as significant blood loss can occur from disconnected or dislodged arterial lines, especially in children.

7. MAINTENANCE AND MONITORING OF THE ADEQUACY OF ANAESTHESIA

N. S. Morton

Monitoring of the adequacy of anaesthesia relies on clinical signs of too light a level of anaesthesia, and specialized electronic brain monitors. The anaesthetist is constantly on the look out for signs of 'lightness' and tries to titrate or match the delivery of anaesthesia to the intensity of the surgical stimulus. Clinical signs are patient movement, tear formation, dilation of the pupils, sweating, increase in heart rate, increase in blood pressure and increase in respiratory rate. It is important to relate these signs to what is happening surgically as there may be other explanations for these signs of 'lightness'. For example, inadequate ventilation with a rise in CO_2 can produce many of these signs!

Electronic monitoring of depth of anaesthesia is in its infancy, with no foolproof simple method currently available. Various versions of processed EEG signals have been tried but are difficult to interpret. More recently, the auditory evoked response (AER) has been used and AER changes do seem to be able to follow changes in the depth of anaesthesia. This technique involves stimulating the eardrum with clicks through small earphones and recording the response of the brain. As the level of anaesthesia deepens, the waveform changes and this change can be measured.

8. Maintenance and Monitoring of the Adequacy of Muscle Relaxation

N. S. Morton

Monitoring of muscle relaxation should be routine whenever a neuromuscular blocking drug is used. This allows the anaesthetist to more accurately assess the effect of a dose of muscle relaxant (i.e. is it producing adequate muscle relaxation for surgery) but also how long a dose lasts, when is another dose needed, when it is safe to reverse the effects of the relaxant and whether reversal is adequate.

These features are important clinically because of wide variation between patients in their responses to a given dose of muscle relaxant, because inadequate relaxation may interfere with ventilation or the surgical procedure, because timing of the need for extra doses of relaxants varies widely between patients, and because inadequate reversal of muscle relaxation is highly dangerous!

The clinical signs of inadequate muscle relaxation are most obviously movement of the patient's limbs, head or facial muscles. Breathing movements of the chest wall and/or the diaphragm may be seen or jerky diaphragmatic movements (hiccoughs) may occur. The abdominal wall muscles may become tight, making access for the surgeon difficult. The inflation pressure on the ventilator may increase because of abdominal muscle tightness or because the patient is trying to breathe against the ventilator.

To monitor neuromuscular transmission, a nerve stimulator can be used to send a current down a nerve to a muscle group and the strength of the response of the muscles can be measured on a graph, by looking or by feeling the 'twitch' of the relevant muscles (Fig. 8.1). The modern nerve stimulator is a compact box of electronics which is usually attached to the patient via two wires and two adhesive skin surface electrodes similar to those used for ECG monitoring. With a stimulus of the correct current as recommended in the manufacturer's data sheet, if there is no response (assuming the machine is working and the electrodes have been applied correctly) then we can say the patient is fully relaxed. By studying a series of four twitches spaced one second apart (the 'train of four'), we can judge the amount of relaxation. If four twitches are present and look and/or feel equally strong then we can say

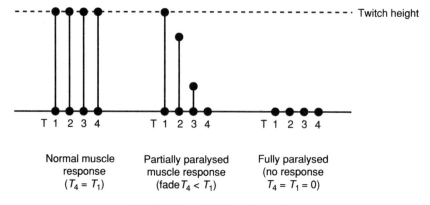

Fig. 8.1 'Train of four' muscle stimulation

the patient is not clinically relaxed at all or fully reversed. Such a patients should be able to breathe well and lift their head up off the pillow to command, provided they are not too sedated. If four twitches are present but the first twitch is stronger than the rest ('fade') it suggests some degree of muscle relaxation is still present. If there are less than four twitches then there is still more of a relaxant effect present. It is not safe to try to reverse a patient until at least one or two of the four twitches is easily seen or felt.

Various other patterns of nerve stimulation are used and some are said to be more sensitive than the 'train of four'.

The important factors affecting the accurate monitoring of muscle relaxation and the effects of relaxants are:

- current applied
- electrode contact
- skin and tissue conductivity
- temperature: hypothermia
- poor peripheral perfusion
- dose of muscle relaxant
- acidosis
- kidney failure
- liver failure
- some volatile anaesthetic agents.

The factors prolonging relaxant effects are:

- enzyme defects, for example pseudocholinesterase deficiency
- increasing dose of muscle relaxant

- some volatile anaesthetic agents
- hypothermia
- acidosis
- kidney failure
- liver failure
- some drugs e.g. aminoglycoside antibiotics such as gentamicin.

9. SAFETY IN THE ANAESTHETIC ROOM AND THEATRE

H. Hosie

Hospitals are potentially dangerous places with potent drugs, potentially dangerous chemicals and electrical and mechanical devices used every day. Transmission of infection to or from patients is another major danger. Anaesthetic rooms, theatres and recovery are areas where safety considerations are essential and should involve three groups of people – your patient, your colleagues and yourself. It is your duty to be aware of local protocols, guidelines and procedures which have been drawn up to comply with recommendations and legislation to ensure safe work practices. Ignorance is no excuse – it is too late to find the fire escape when the theatre is in flames!

THE ENVIRONMENT IN GENERAL

Anaesthetic rooms, theatres and recovery areas should be clean, comfortable and tidy. Certain areas will be designated sterile, some clean and some dirty. Strict observation of these areas will reduce the risk of infection in patients and staff. Chemicals used in cleaning or maintaining sterility must be correctly handled as some may be toxic. Each hospital should have policies which clearly outline the procedures involved in handling these chemicals in line with Control of Substances Hazardous to Health (COSHH) recommendations and in conjunction with the local Occupational Health Service. All personnel working in the theatre environment should be aware of these policies and their impact on practice.

The temperature and humidity of the theatre area should also be strictly controlled, partly for the staff who work there, but more importantly, for the comfort and safety of the patient. In specialized areas there may be adjustments in temperature and humidity. For instance, in paediatric anaesthesia, particularly neonatal anaesthesia, the temperature must be kept high to prevent heat loss from the infant. Conversely in some theatres, such as cardiac surgery or neurosurgery, such high temperatures are inappropriate and the patient may be actively cooled.

General tidiness is important in the complicated surroundings in the operating theatre, with sophisticated equipment, trailing cables, pipelines and box upon box of sterile disposables. Equipment should be kept in a specific site and tidied away after every use to minimize damage. Repair and replacement costs are high and lost components lead to delays and inefficiency. It is your responsibility to ensure 'good housekeeping' practices at work.

A considerable amount of waste is produced in the theatre area from disposables, sterile supplies and single-use equipment. Some of this will be contaminated with blood, secretions or other body fluids and should be incinerated. Lots of waste is clean, however, and can be disposed of in a conventional way. Items such as sharps and needles must always be disposed of in suitable protective containers. It is the responsibility of all who work in the theatre environment to dispose of contaminated and waste products safely and sensibly. Each hospital should have its own guidelines or protocols for the management and disposal of hazardous or infected waste. These should be scrutinized and memorized.

THE ENVIRONMENT IN PARTICULAR

The Anaesthetic Room and Equipment

Before use all anaesthetic machines and gas supplies should be checked according to the checklist issued by the Association of Anaesthetists (see Ch. 2). Ensuring the correct gas supplies involves the use of the oxygen analyser, which should be calibrated daily. Attaching the correct gas cylinder to the correct yoke is ensured by the pin index system and the colour coding system of cylinders. Piped gas supplies should be guaranteed as each pipeline will only fit into the appropriately colour-coded noninterchangeable Schrader valve connector. Accidents have been known to occur when servicing pipelines, however resulting in misconnections. Broken pins or missing Bodok seals on cylinders can result in misconnection or leaks. The oxygen analyser remains the gold standard safety monitor of oxygen supply.

Modern anaesthetic vaporizers also have safety features. Each vaporizer is specific for a specific vapour. If a different vapour is used the concentration of vapour dialled up using the vaporizer dial will be inaccurate due to the physical differences between vapours. Attempts to ensure that the correct vapour is poured into the appropriate vaporizer involve the use of colour-coded 'keyed' vaporizer fillers. Each plastic filler will only fit into one type of vaporizer and one type of vapour bottle. However, accidents have occurred when the vapour bottle has had a different vapour or liquid decanted into it. This practice must not be permitted in your theatre.

Modern anaesthesia uses many different monitors to assess the patient's condition. These monitors are usually electrically powered, either through mains electricity or batteries. Mains electricity is susceptible to power surges and although much equipment is 'shielded' from the effects of the surges, accidents have occurred when power surges have possibly corrupted the microchips within the monitors or equipment. Most hospitals today have strict controls over the use of mobile phones within intensive care units and theatres because of the problem of electronic interference. Monitors and equipment such as syringe pumps, heating blankets and IV fluid warmers must be carefully checked to ensure accurate performance. Registers should be kept on every 'medical device', which should ensure a full history of each piece of equipment, including servicing history and reported faults or damage. Those who use these medical devices must be aware of Hazard Warnings or Safety Bulletins affecting any devices in use in their clinical area.

When using monitors such as ECGs, pulse oximeters, automatic sphygmo-manometers and gas analysers always check that alarms are set and are appropriate for that patient.

The responsibility of handling and preparing drugs for administration is a heavy one. Medico-legal practice frequently encounters errors in prescription and administration. If you prepare or administer drugs certain rules should be followed. Drugs should be prepared according to local guidelines, be clearly labelled and kept in a clean or sterile tray. Ampoules must be checked for drug name, strength and date of expiry. Syringes must be clearly labelled with the drug name and strength. Drugs which are not used or are discarded should be disposed of appropriately and in the case of controlled drugs should be entered on the controlled drug register. Administration of intra-venous drugs should be covered by local protocols. Be aware of and fulfil the training requirements for these protocols.

Intravenous access should be secured in all patients. Cannulae must be inserted using a clean or aseptic technique, careful secured and documented. Intra-arterial lines must be clearly marked as such, and clearly documented so that no drugs are inadvertently given by that route. Drugs given intravenously may cause occasional thrombophlebitis; drugs given intra-arterially cause intense arterial spasm and may cause irreversible ischaemia of the limb distal to the artery, ultimately resulting in amputation. Epidural catheters should only be inserted under aseptic techniques as should other catheters or central venous cannulae. They too should be adequately secured and clearly marked and documented. Epidural cannulae are conventionally marked with a yellow sticker, central venous lines with blue stickers and arterial lines in red. This is to prevent accidental injection or infusion of drugs by the wrong route.

Laryngeal masks and tracheal tubes must be adequately secured and if a throat pack is used, the fact should be communicated to the person scrubbed, who should add it their swab count and clearly record it.

The Theatre

Anaesthetized patients cannot protect themselves so the greatest care should be taken to protect joints and limbs from overflexion or overextension. Adequate padding must be used to protect nerves and limbs from pressure injuries and the patient must be adequately secured. If diathermy is used the plate must be attached to a suitable site, not overlying metal implants or prostheses. It is beyond the scope of this book to enumerate all the potentials for damage to patients. It is a salutary lesson, however, to read some of the medical defence societies reports. Reports have been made of instances of corneal scarring from wrongly taping eyes which were not properly closed to burning of digits in neonates monitored with pulse oximeter probes which got too hot.

In some theatres, X-rays or screening techniques are used to confirm the position of probes, needles, plates, prostheses or bones. Personnel must ensure that appropriate lead shielding devices are available not only for the theatre staff but also for the patient. In work areas where radiation exposure is frequent, measurement devices to record the exposure of the personnel may be used.

The risks of explosion and burning have always existed in the theatre area. There is a risk of explosion when opening a high pressure cylinder or where oxygen is being used and there is an ignitable source of material. Lasers may raise the temperature of materials such as plastic endotracheal tubes so that they start to burn. In the oxygen-rich atmosphere the subsequent fire can cause much damage. Fires involving alcohol-based cleaning fluids, faulty diathermy cables, foil heat-retaining drapes, lasers, anaesthetic gases and many others have all been reported. All equipment in theatre must be used carefully with particular attention to electrical safety, ignition and explosion hazards.

Static electricity is another possible source of ignition, although it is much less of a problem with modern anaesthetic gases.

Protection of Self

Some of the restrictions on personal dress and decoration in theatre must seem petty. However, you have responsibility to yourself, your colleagues and your patients to maintain a safe environment. This means that your appearance should be clean, neat and tidy and that theatre garb is kept clean and uncontaminated as far as is possible. Protective clothing such as plastic gloves, goggles and gowns may be indicated in all or some cases. The use of facemasks may be insisted upon in some theatre areas and not in others. It is sensible to cover any cuts, sores or grazes partly to protect yourself and partly to protect others. Consideration must be given to obtaining immunization against some blood-borne viruses such as hepatitis. This will be insisted upon by employing authorities and advice should be sought either from your general medical practitioner or from the Occupational Health Service.

Protection of Patient

Protection of the patient starts as soon as you accept the care of the patient from the ward nurse. The patient's identity, consent and operation, including site and side, should be confirmed, as should any other relevant information on the theatre checklist. Throughout anaesthesia, surgery and recovery you must protect the patient from potential harm and damage as they are unable to protect themselves. By consenting to an operation they are placing their trust in you and you have a responsibility to treat and protect then as you would wish for yourself or one of your family. Respect for the patient's wishes must be considered but the safety of the patient is paramount.

Positioning of the patient

The position of the patient during anaesthesia and surgery depends on the needs of the surgeon for access to a part of the body and the needs of the anaesthetist for the safe conduct of the anaesthesia. Gravity affects the circulation and lung function. Blood pools in the legs if the patient is head up. In the head down position, or with the legs raised, venous blood return to the heart is improved. When the patient lies on their back the diaphragm is pushed up by the contents of the abdomen. This makes the rear half of the diaphragm work more efficiently when the patient is awake causing better ventilation of the dependent (posterior) segments of the lung which matches up with the better blood flow to these same areas. When the patient is anaesthetised, the diaphragm moves up even more and basal areas of lung tend to collapse. This is counteracted to some extent when ventilation is controlled.

The principles of safe patient positioning are to avoid overstretching joints, avoid forcing limbs into particular positions, to provide adequate padding for pressure points and to coordinate movement of the anaesthetised patient into the required position. Joint dislocation, nerve damage due to stretching or direct pressure or muscle damage can occur.

The lithotomy position is used frequently in gynaecology, urology, and colorectal surgery. The legs are flexed at the hips and spread to allow access. The legs must be held carefully while they are both put into position at the same time. Vertical bars attached to the operating table must be secured firmly and either have padded supports behind the knees or slings to hold the feet. It is important that padding is placed between the supports and the calf to prevent nerve or muscle damage or diathermy burns. The arms may be placed by the side or out from the body on arm support boards but should not be at an angle of more than 90° because the brachial plexus can be over-stretched and damaged. Any encircling straps on legs or arms must not be too tight in case venous or arterial blood flow is occluded.

The lateral position is commonly used for thoracic surgery and sometimes for orthopaedic, plastic, or neurosurgery. The arm positioning and padding of arms and legs is extremely important to protect against nerve, muscle, and skin pressure damage and stretching injuries.

The prone position is used for back surgery, rectal procedures and for excision of lesions or for skin grafting in burns. A pillow is usually placed under the hips and upper chest to keep the abdomen free which helps the diaphragm to descend and improves ventilation. Padding around the face, eye protection, tracheal tube security, vascular line fixation and pressure area protection are vital in this position. The arm position can be by the side or the arms may be placed flexed at shoulder and elbow so the hands are beside the head. Care must be taken to avoid shoulder dislocation and overstretching of the brachial plexus.

A variant of the prone position is the 'knee-elbow' position which is used for back surgery. A special frame device is used to maintain this position and the same principles of positioning apply.

KEY LEARNING POINTS

1. Clinical signs are the best early monitors of an obstructed airway or inadequate ventilation.

2. Electronic monitors of oxygenation, carbon dioxide output and anaesthetic agent concentration are vital for patient safety.

3. When ventilation is controlled, additional electronic monitoring is essential to ensure the correct volumes, pressures, oxygen delivery and carbon dioxide output are maintained.

4. Minimum circulatory monitoring comprises clinical signs of good perfusion, regular non-invasive blood pressure measurement and continuous ECG and pulse oximetry display. Continuous arterial, venous and pulmonary pressure monitoring are used in major cases as appropriate.

5. Whenever a muscle relaxant is used it is advisable to monitor its effects with a peripheral nerve stimulator to allow titration of dosage and adequacy of reversal.

6. Depth of anaesthesia is judged clinically at present but monitors are being developed to give more accurate assessments.

7. Safety measures must be given a high priority in the potentially hazardous operating theatre environment to protect patients and personnel.

Further Reading

'Ward's Anaesthetic Equipment', 3rd edition. A Davey, JTB Moyle, CS Ward. WB Saunders Company Ltd, London, 1992.

'Understanding Anaesthesia', 3rd edition. LES Carrie, PJ Simpson, MT Popat. Butterworth-Heinemann, Oxford, 1996.

'Practical procedures in anaesthesia and critical care'. PJF Baskett, A Dow, J Nolan, K Maull. Mosby, London, 1995.

Cucchiara RF, Faust RJ. Patient positioning. In: Anaesthesia. 4th edition. Edited by R. D. Miller. Churchill Livingstone, New York. 1994. p. 1057–1074.

Relevance

ODP Level 3   Units 3, 5, 6, 8.

SECTION 4
EMERGENCIES IN ANAESTHESIA

Emergencies don't happen often but they occur unpredictably. They may happen at induction, during surgery and in the recovery area. Anaesthetists often refer to such events as critical incidents – that is something that happens which could do harm to the patient if not properly recognized and treated. This is one area where skilled assistance is of vital importance. Remember too that an assistant may have more experience of these situations than a trainee anaesthetist and that appropriate action on your part may save the patient's life.

It is clear that the anaesthetist is ultimately responsible for checking equipment and drugs which are likely to be needed for emergencies but the assistant is vitally important as often they will be delegated to bring these items to the patient quickly while the anaesthetist starts resuscitation.

Good assistants will always anticipate emergencies. For instance, if the anaesthetist has chosen to use a local anaesthetic block as part of his technique, the good anaesthetist and assistant will have checked and know where drugs used to treat local anaesthetic toxicity are kept. In addition to checking the anaesthetic machine, a good assistant will familiarize themself with the location of the cardiac arrest box, emergency intubation equipment, nearest defibrillator and Ambu bag. Many theatre suites have all equipment stored in mirror image cupboards, but not all do. If you are moved to a different theatre it is vital that you know where all the equipment is.

Things you should know:

- where the cardiac arrest box is stored
- where the adrenaline is stored and in what concentration
- where drugs used in emergencies are kept
- where tracheal tubes and connectors are to hand (in all sizes)
- where an Ambu bag is stored
- where the nearest defibrillator is located
- how to tilt the trolley
- how to tilt the bed
- where you can get hold of blood bottles and forms
- the location of portable suction.

Above all BE PREPARED.

10. AIRWAY

H. Hosie, N. S. Morton

AIRWAY OBSTRUCTION AND LARYNGOSPASM

As noted in Section 3 the early warning signs of airway obstruction are clinical, especially when the patient is breathing spontaneously. Monitors become more important as more invasive techniques are used to maintain the airway, so that in the intubated patient whose ventilation is being controlled, monitors give vital early warning signs.

In any case of airway obstruction, it is very important to make the diagnosis early and to intervene safely to secure the airway. As noted before, this is because airway obstruction will usually lead to hypoxia (low PaO_2), hypercarbia (high $PaCO_2$), lightening of the level of anaesthesia and increased risk of regurgitation and aspiration of stomach contents.

Some patients have evidence of airway obstruction detected at the preoperative assessment, for example due to tumours or infections, and extreme care and skill is needed to deal with such cases. The difficult airway is dealt with in Chapter 3.

Airway obstruction developing during anaesthesia is an emergency and intervention should be rapid and decisive. First the anaesthetist should ask the surgeon to stop the operation. This is because surgical stimulation with too light a level of anaesthesia is a common trigger for laryngeal spasm. Remember if the airway is obstructed, the spontaneously breathing patient will tend to lighten so continuing the surgical stimulation will make matters worse.

Secondly the anaesthetist should switch to 100% oxygen, ensure a good seal with the facemask, use the triple manoeuvre (jaw thrust) to pull the jaw forward and ensure the mouth is open. This may be all that is needed and after increasing the depth of anaesthesia, surgery can proceed. The assistant should prepare to help with tracheal intubation. An oropharyngeal or nasopharyngeal airway may help but only if the patient is deeply enough asleep to tolerate one. If airway obstruction is not relieved at once by these simple manoeuvres in the unintubated patient, then assume laryngospasm has occurred and the anaesthetist will proceed at once to give suxamethonium with or without atropine. Immediately the suxamethonium has taken effect, the airway should clear enabling ventilation with 100% oxygen by mask. The airway is then secured with a tracheal tube as appropriate. Beware of regurgitation in this situation as it is a common accompaniment to laryngospasm and indeed may be the *cause* of the spasm in some cases.

It is obvious that this sequence must be carried out very quickly and so suxamethonium, atropine, laryngoscopes, tracheal tubes and airways must be immediately to hand and venous access immediately available for such a situation. For *every* anaesthetic, this should be routine, whatever the age, medical state and surgical procedure.

For the patient with a laryngeal mask airway (LMA) in place the same applies because laryngospasm can occur in such cases. Most anaesthetists remove the LMA at an early stage as it may have triggered laryngospasm and follow the same sequence noted above.

The LMA is a very helpful device but can cause a set of problems which lead to obstruction of the airway. The epiglottis can be pushed down ahead of the device and obstruct the laryngeal inlet. The LMA opening may not be properly aligned with the larynx either because it is in too far, not in far enough or is rotated. The LMA may be kinked or obstructed by secretions. If the cuff is overinflated, it may bulge or herniate into the larynx causing airway obstruction.

In the intubated patient, the airway is more secure but obstruction of the airway can still occur. The tube itself may be blocked, kinked or malpositioned. An overinflated cuff can obstruct the end of the tube. It is as important to make a correct diagnosis in the intubated patient to sort out whether the tube is obstructed, positioned wrongly or the airway obstruction is further down the respiratory tract. When in doubt most anaesthetists take the tube out and replace it but simpler measures such as passage of a catheter to suction the tube or a small saline lavage to clear secretions or blood may be all that is needed. Again it is obvious that all the equipment to allow these manoeuvres must be ready immediately to hand in case they are needed and the assistant must be prepared for all these unexpected situations at all times.

REGURGITATION AND ASPIRATION OF STOMACH CONTENTS

This is the movement of stomach contents up the gullet (oesophagus), into the pharynx and through the larynx into the trachea, bronchi and lungs. For regurgitation to occur there must be stomach contents present. Usually liquid contents empty relatively quickly from the stomach, while solid food has to be broken down first and takes longer. Food with a high fat content takes longest of all. Remember milk becomes a solid high in fat content when it enters the stomach. There is an assumption that a period of 4 to 6 hours fasting will ensure an empty stomach and that may be the case in some patients. However, in patients with a history of gastric or duodenal ulcers or of gastric surgery this may not be true. Patients who are in pain or have been involved in trauma will also have slowed transit times through the stomach, as will patients who have been given opioid painkillers such as morphine.

Normally, there is no regurgitation of stomach contents into the lower oesophagus because the muscle at the lower end of the oesophagus is closed partly due to contraction of the oesophageal muscle and partly because of loops of muscle from the diaphragm constrict this area and keep it shut. The area is known as the lower oesophageal sphincter (LOS). In some people the LOS is ineffective and they often complain of heartburn when the acid stomach contents wash into the unprotected lower oesophageal lining. People who are particularly at risk are pregnant women, people with hiatus hernia, very fat individuals and those with tumours in the abdomen or who have obstructed bowel.

In the awake person regurgitation of gastric contents can occur but they will not aspirate the contents across the larynx. Reflexes such as the gag reflex prevent this by closing the laryngeal inlet tightly against any fluid and causing coughing. The anaesthetized patient has lost these protective reflexes and cannot protect his airway – thus aspiration into the airways and lungs may occur.

There are two main problems with aspirating or inhaling stomach contents.

Inhalation of Food Debris

If the patient inhales bits of food they can block the trachea, the main bronchi or the smaller conducting bronchi. In the event of a piece of food blocking the trachea no gas exchange can take place until it is removed. It may be possible to remove the debris visually via a laryngoscope and forceps or suction. It may, however, be impossible and the airway must be maintained until formal rigid bronchoscopy can take place. This may necessitate a tracheostomy beyond the obstruction or the use of a minitracheostomy. Other solutions include insertion of cannulae via the cricothyroid membrane but the basic idea is to get oxygen into the lungs beyond the obstructing debris.

If the blockage is lower down then oxygen can at least get into one lung even if the other main bronchus is blocked. Bronchoscopy is usually needed to remove the debris and may be technically very difficult as debris often sets up a very powerful inflammatory reaction in the lining of the airways.

Inhalation of Liquid Contents

The contents of the stomach are usually very acid. Because they are liquid, droplets can spread quite far down the airway to the alveoli of the lungs. The acid damages the alveolar membrane making it thick and swollen and can impair transport of oxygen across the alveolar membrane into the blood. This can give rise to the acid aspiration syndrome, which has a high mortality and necessitates ventilation with high concentrations of oxygen.

Prevention is by the following methods:

- fasting patients (6 h solids and milk, 4 h breast milk, 3 h clear fluids)
- identifying 'at risk' patients
- treating 'at risk' patients with antacids such as socium citrate and H_2 receptor antagonists such as cimetidine or ranitidine
- rapid sequence induction.

What to do if the patient regurgitates:

1. Tip the trolley
2. suction the patient
3. keep cricoid pressure on.

Remember to tip the trolley and perform suction with one hand while maintaining cricoid pressure with the other. You must have the patient on a tipping trolley, the right way round and you must know how to tip the trolley and activate the suction apparatus, which should have been checked to ensure that it works.

11. BREATHING

H. Hosie, N. S. Morton

RESPIRATORY ARREST

Respiratory arrest or apnoea is the cessation of breathing. Breathing is controlled by the respiratory centre, which is found in the brainstem. There are three separate areas of function, the inspiratory centre, the pneumotaxic centre and the expiratory centre. In normal inspiration (breathing in) there is increasing electrical activity in the inspiratory centre. Nervous impulses are conducted along the phrenic and intercostal nerves and cause contraction of the diaphragm and sometimes the intercostal muscles. This causes a negative intrathroacic pressure, air enters and expands the lungs. As the lungs stretch and expand, stretch receptors are activated which send impulses to the pneumotaxic centre. This inhibits the inspiratory centre and stops further expansion of the lungs. Normally air is then expelled passively with the elastic recoil of the lung tissue. Occasionally the expiratory centre becomes active, contracting expiratory muscles and causing air to be blown out. The inspiratory centre is the area of the brain initiating inspiration and it responds principally to changes in the hydrogen ion concentration (H^+) of the cerebrospinal fluid (CSF). The hydrogen ion concentration of CSF reflects the concentration of carbon dioxide in the blood – as the carbon dioxide level rises, so does the H^+ concentration. This activates the respiratory centre to increase ventilation and more carbon dioxide is expired. Drugs or diseases affecting the brainstem or phrenic nerves will cause apnoea. The respiratory centre in the brain may be affected by many drugs used in anaesthetic practice, especially the induction agents, opioids and benzodiazepines. It may also be damaged as a result of trauma, haemorrhage or tumour.

Similarly the muscles supplied by the phrenic and intercostal nerves (the diaphragm and intercostal muscles) must be in good working order. Failure of these muscles to contract adequately is the peripheral cause of respiratory arrest. The respiratory muscles will be affected by muscle relaxants and by disease states such as myasthenia or motor neurone disease.

Signs and Symptoms

At respiratory arrest there is no chest movement, there are no breath sounds on auscultation and there is no misting of humid expired air on the face mask, LMA or tracheal tube. The arrest may be preceded by a slowing respiratory rate. Cyanosis may be seen and the pulse oximeter will show a fall in saturation although if supplementary oxygen is being given this may be delayed. If the patient has a laryngeal mask or tracheal tube in place the capnograph will show no expiratory trace. This can also happen when the sampling tube is kinked or blocked, but if the apnoea alarm sounds on the capnograph check the patency of the airway and respiratory movements first before checking the machine. Spirometry detects the movement of gas. It will detect low tidal volumes or low minute volumes but is restricted to use with either the laryngeal mask or endotracheal tube. It is not normally used with facemasks as there are too many leaks for accuracy. Some machines have been developed as apnoea alarms for use in recovery, especially with opiate infusions. Most depend upon movement of gas or detection of carbon dioxide. This is limiting as close fitting face masks are needed, which patients find difficult to tolerate, and the frequency of false alarms is high.

Treatment

Oxygen must be available either from an anaesthetic machine, piped gas or cylinder. In the case of cylinders, spanners must always be attached and ready to switch on. A method of administering oxygen under pressure is also necessary. The Ambubag device is very useful particularly with the oxygen enrichment reservoir. If no artificial airway is in place an oral or pharyngeal airway may be useful and intermittent positive pressure ventilation started using a bag and mask. Oxygen at flows in excess of estimated minute volume should be given and preparations for intubation made.

Drugs

Drugs which may be used in respiratory arrest secondary to central causes fall into two main categories – specific drug antagonists and respiratory stimulants.

Drugs antagonists are 'antidotes' to certain specific drugs. Pharmacologically they bind to the same receptor proteins on the target tissue as the drug but they have no pharmacological effect. In this way they stop the drug binding to the receptor protein and so prevent the effect.

Naloxone is a specific antagonist for all the opiate drugs. As it bind to the same receptor protein as the opiates it stops opiate-induced respiratory depression and also reverses the painkiller, sedative and euphoric effects of the opiates. It is available in 1 ml ampoules containing 400 μg of the drug. A standard dose would be 200–400 μg in an adult patient. Its effect is short lived, lasting about 20 min and in some patients the dose may need to be repeated or given an infusion.

Flumazenil is a specific benzodiazepine antagonist and will reverse the sedative effects of all benzodiazepines in a similar fashion. It is available in a 5 ml ampoule containing 500 μg. A standard adult dose would be 200 μg (2 ml) with further 100 μg) 1 ml) increments to a maximum of 1 mg (10 ml). Again its action is short lived. It may need to be repeated or given by infusion.

The only respiratory stimulant in common use is doxapram. This drug works by stimulating the peripheral chemoreceptors and causes an increase mainly in tidal volume and minute volume. It has a lesser effect on respiratory rate. It is available in a 5 ml ampoule containing 100 mg and also in a 500 ml bag of 5% dextrose containing 1 g doxapram. The bag is sometimes used for infusions in patients with respiratory failure. A standard adult dose is 70–100 mg. Side-effects include anxiety, wakefulness and agitation. As it has central effects, at high dosages it can cause hypertension, tachycardia and muscle fasciculations, but these are rarely seen following a single dose in the recovery room situation.

Respiratory arrest secondary to peripheral causes is due to weakness of the respiratory musculature. In disease states such as myasthenia, supportive ventilation is instituted until the effects of muscle relaxants have worn off. In other diseases states muscle function can be optimized by ensuring adequate plasma concentrations of calcium and phosphate salts. In normal patients with good respiratory muscle function apnoea may be due to inadequate reversal of the neuromuscular blockers.

Muscles contract following a nervous impulse which releases a neurotransmitter substance – acetylcholine. This transmitter binds to receptor sites on the muscle and activates a chain of events which ultimately causes a muscle contraction. Neuromuscular relaxants usually work by competing with acetylcholine to bind on the receptor sites. When lots of neuromuscular blocker is available just after an injection of muscle relaxant, almost all the receptor sites are occupied by blocker and the muscle cannot contract. Neuromuscular blockers, will, in time, be broken down by the body but usually at the end of the operation reversal agents are given. Neostigmine stops the acetyclcholine naturally produced by the nerves from being broken down. This means that the concentration of acetylcholine is increased, acetylcholine binds to more receptors and the muscle is able to contract. As neostigmine is not specific for the neuromuscular junction it has effects at other sites where acetylcholine is a neurotransmitter. Because of this neostigmine is given in combination with atropine or glycopyrrolate which block potentially serious side-effects of neostigmine, such as slowing of the heart.

The effects of neuromuscular blockers can be prolonged in patients who have difficulty in metabolizing (breaking down) the drug. Some relaxants are metabolized to inactive chemicals by the liver, some by the kidney and some by enzymes usually present in many tissues. The effects of the relaxant can be prolonged when patients have liver problems, kidney problems or in a few people who have a genetic inability to produce the pseudocholinesterase activity. If these problems are recognized preoperatively the anaesthetist will select a relaxant which will not have prolonged effects but this is occasionally not recognized preoperatively. Residual neuromuscular blockade may present as apnoea and can be diagnosed using a peripheral nerve stimulator and in some cases by blood testing.

HYPOXAEMIA

Hypoxaemia means that there is too little oxygen reaching the body tissues. It can occur for a variety of reasons. There must be enough oxygen in the gases being breathed, this oxygen must be able to get into the lungs and must be able to transfer across from lungs to blood and be carried in adequate amounts to the tissues. The tissues must then be capable of using the oxygen. If any of these steps fails then tissue hypoxia occurs (Table 11.1).

Arterial blood gas and pH samples confirm the low oxygen in arterial blood and acidosis (a low pH) often accompanies hypoxaemia.

Table 11.1

STEPS IN OXYGEN SUPPLY	EXAMPLE OF FAILURE
1. Oxygen in inspired air	Cylinder/pipeline problems; smoke inhalation
2. Breathing	Respiratory depression; apnoea, airway obstruction
3. Transfer from lungs to blood	Lung fibrosis; severe respiratory disease
4. Carriage by blood	Circulatory failure, shock, abnormal haemoglobins, carbon monoxide poisoning
5. Use by tissues	Poisoning, for example cyanide in smoke inhalation

The treatment varies somewhat with the cause, but 100% oxygen should be given at once and ventilation assisted or controlled until a more definitive diagnosis of the cause is made. Check oxygen sources, adequacy of the patency of the airway, breathing and adequacy of the circulation (i.e. the ABC of resuscitation).

In certain cases, specific treatments can be given by the anaesthetist, for example antidotes to sedatives or opioids; or methylene blue for methaemoglobinaemia.

BRONCHOSPASM

Bronchospasm describes the narrowing of small airways in the lungs and is most commonly seen as a response to an irritant in the lungs, as part of a response to an allergy, and in asthma or respiratory infections.

Irritants include toxic gases or smoke, dry or cold gases, acid or solid food particles from the stomach, or an endotracheal tube, especially if it is too long and touches the carina at the junction of the right and left main bronchi.

As part of an allergic reaction to a drug, fluid or substance such as latex, large amounts of histamine and other chemical mediators are produced which can cause bronchospasm (see Chapter 13).

In asthma, the patient's airways are irritable and prone to spasm, especially if they are instrumented or exposed to noxious stimuli from the stress of surgery. Light levels of anaesthesia in the asthmatic subjected to a surgical stimulus are very likely to induce bronchospasm.

Respiratory infections due to bacteria or viruses make the larynx and airways very irritable and it is unwise to anaesthetize such patients unless it is absolutely essential.

Management by the anaesthetist of bronchospasm occurring during anaesthesia comprises stopping the trigger, deepening the level of anaesthesia, increasing the inspired oxygen concentration, giving bronchodilators and steroids. In those with respiratory infections who have to have an anaesthetic, atropine can be helpful as some of the bronchospasm is due to overactivity of the vagal nerve supply to the airways.

For treatment of anaphylaxis see Chapter 13.

PNEUMOTHORAX

A pneumothorax is when an air leak occurs from the lung surface or from an airway. The air usually tracks into the space between the chest wall and lung surface. The lung tends to collapse and the air leak tends to worsen, especially if the patient is being ventilated. The air pocket enlarges and eventually becomes under tension, compressing the lung and the venous return to the heart. This is a life-threatening emergency and the tension within the chest cavity must be relieved at once. A needle or cannula can be inserted as an immediate measure. A formal chest drain is then inserted and connected to an underwater seal system to definitively drain the air pocket. The assistant must know the location of the equipment for chest drainage, including the chest drainage tubes and underwater seal devices. Most operating theatres and intensive care units have a trolley or set for emergency chest drain insertion. An air leak may continue for some time, depending on the underlying cause.

Patients at particular risk of pneumothroax are those with lung disease, where high airway pressures have been used, those who have received chest trauma or blast injuries, or where central venous lines have been inserted by the jugular or subclavian routes.

12. CIRCULATION

H. Hosie

CARDIAC ARREST IN ADULTS

Cardiac arrest is the cessation of pump action by the heart. This leads to cessation of blood flow to all organs and most importantly the brain. Cessation of blood flow to the brain for 3 min or more will result in hypoxic brain damage in normal circumstances. Recognition of cardiac arrest, prompt treatment of the underlying cause, if possible, and effective cardiopulmonary resuscitation is vital.

Cardiac muscle differs from other muscle fibres in that the fibres contract rhythmically without needing a nervous impulse to initiate contraction. That is why transplanted hearts can beat without a nerve supply. Certain specialized areas of heart muscle contain pacemaker fibres and conduction fibres. These areas also contract rhythmically but at a faster rate than other areas and they cause the atria and ventricles to contract sequentially so that as the atria contract they push blood into the ventricles which then contract pushing blood into the pulmonary artery or the aorta and so send blood to all the tissues of the body. The nerve supply to the heart is part of the autonomic nervous system and is made up of the cardiac sympathetic fibres, originating from the thoracic part of the spinal cord and which speed the heart up, and the parasympathetic vagal fibres, which arise from the 10th cranial nerve and tend to slow the heart's innate rate.

It can be seen then, that if the ventricles fail to contract, or if they don't fill up with blood properly, the blood flow following ventricular contraction stops. Cardiac arrest occurs with three underlying rhythm disturbances:

1. asystole when contraction stops
2. ventricular fibrillation when the ventricles contract very rapidly at 150–200 times per min in a disorganised fashion which produces no pumping action and thus no pulse
3. electromechanical dissociation when, although electrical activity continues, the ventricles do not contract at all and there is no pulse.

Signs and Symptoms

Because blood is not flowing to the tissues the initial signs and symptoms of cardiac arrest are loss of consciousness, loss of palpable pulse and respiratory arrest. The patient looks pale or sometimes blue and cyanosed. Pulse oximeter reading will fail or may show desaturation. An ECG will show one of the three rhythm disturbances: asystole; (a flat trace) ventricular fibrillation (chaotic waves) or electromechanical dissociation (complexes, no pulse).

Treatment

The aim of cardiopulmonary resuscitation is to obtain an adequate blood flow to the tissues by external cardiac massage and ensure that the blood should be adequately oxygenated by artificial ventilation. By these methods adequate oxygen should be delivered to the brain to prevent hypoxic brain damage. Treatment of the underlying rhythm disturbance to convert to normal sinus rhythm is the second aim of treatment. Guidelines for basic and advanced life support have been issued by the European Resuscitation Council and are reproduced here. (Fig. 12.1) These must be learnt 'by heart' by all members of the theatre team as there may be needed at any time.

Initially a precordial thump should be given. Many patients will be connected to an ECG and a diagnosis of the rhythm made immediately. In cases of ventricular fibrillation electrical defibrillation is the treatment of choice. If the rhythm is not known defibrillation should be carried out. Intubation and ventilation with 100% oxygen should be performed immediately and intravenous access established. If intubation of i.v. access is going to take too long or the staff are inexperienced, hand ventilation with bag and mask will do initially whilst the first 'loop' of compression/ventilation is started. Each sequence of compression/ventilation is mae up of five compressions of the chest to one ventilated breath.

Treatment consists of defibrillation, initially at 200 J, then at 360 J at sequences of 10 cycles. Drug treatment is initially adrenaline 1 mg but may also include atropine 3 mg, calcium salts, pressor agents such as isoprenaline, adrenaline and noradrenaline and alkalizing agents such as molar sodium bicarbonate (8.4%). All drugs needed at an arrest should be available on a cardiac arrest tray and it is your responsibility to ensure that you know the location of the tray and a defibrillator at any site where anaesthesia may be carried out.

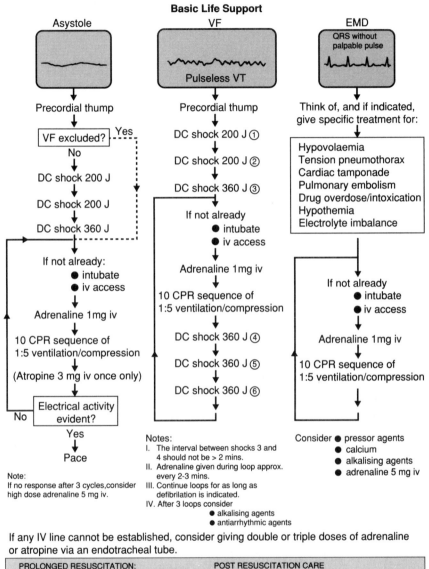

Basic Life Support

Asystole

Precordial thump

VF excluded? — Yes

No

DC shock 200 J

DC shock 200 J

DC shock 360 J

If not already:
● intubate
● iv access

Adrenaline 1mg iv

10 CPR sequence of
1:5 ventilation/compression

(Atropine 3 mg iv once only)

Electrical activity evident?

No — Yes

Pace

Note:
If no response after 3 cycles, consider high dose adrenaline 5 mg iv.

VF

Pulseless VT

Precordial thump

DC shock 200 J ①

DC shock 200 J ②

DC shock 360 J ③

If not already
● intubate
● iv access

Adrenaline 1mg iv

10 CPR sequence of
1:5 ventilation/compression

DC shock 360 J ④

DC shock 360 J ⑤

DC shock 360 J ⑥

Notes:
I. The interval between shocks 3 and 4 should not be > 2 mins.
II. Adrenaline given during loop approx. every 2-3 mins.
III. Continue loops for as long as defibrilation is indicated.
IV. After 3 loops consider
● alkalising agents
● antiarrhythmic agents

EMD

QRS without palpable pulse

Think of, and if indicated, give specific treatment for:

Hypovolaemia
Tension pneumothorax
Cardiac tamponade
Pulmonary embolism
Drug overdose/intoxication
Hypothemia
Electrolyte imbalance

If not already
● intubate
● iv access

Adrenaline 1mg iv

10 CPR sequence of
1:5 ventilation/compression

Consider ● pressor agents
● calcium
● alkalising agents
● adrenaline 5 mg iv

If any IV line cannot be established, consider giving double or triple doses of adrenaline or atropine via an endotracheal tube.

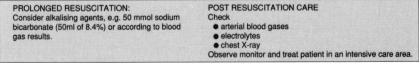

PROLONGED RESUSCITATION:
Consider alkalising agents, e.g. 50 mmol sodium bicarbonate (50ml of 8.4%) or according to blood gas results.

POST RESUSCITATION CARE
Check
● arterial blood gases
● electrolytes
● chest X-ray
Observe monitor and treat patient in an intensive care area.

Fig. 12.1 Adult advanced cardiac life support

CARDIAC ARREST IN CHILDREN

See ERC protocol. (Fig. 12.2) Cardiac arrest in children is nearly always secondary to hypoxaemia. Oxygen and adrenaline are the two most useful drugs in paediatric resuscitation. Ensure airway, oxygenation and ventilation

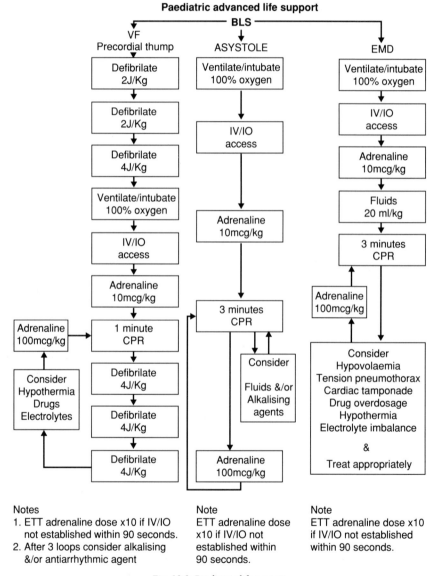

Paediatric advanced life support

Notes
1. ETT adrenaline dose x10 if IV/IO not established within 90 seconds.
2. After 3 loops consider alkalising &/or antiarrhythmic agent

Note
ETT adrenaline dose x10 if IV/IO not established within 90 seconds.

Note
ETT adrenaline dose x10 if IV/IO not established within 90 seconds.

Fig. 12.2 Paediatric life support

are optimal. Cardiac massage at 100 cycles per minute with 20 breaths per minute is usually adequate. High dose adrenaline has been shown to improve outcome. Where venous access is difficult an intraosseous needle placed just below the knee into the marrow cavity of the tibia is quick, effective, and safe for administration of resuscitation drugs and fluids.

Hypotension (Low Blood Pressure)

Hypotension is defined as a persistently low arterial pressure. Arterial blood pressure is expressed in terms of systolic pressure (the peak pressure caused by contraction of the left ventricle of the heart), diastolic pressure (the pressure in the arterial system during diastole when the left ventricle is relaxed) and the mean arterial pressure, which is arithmetically calculated from the systolic and diastolic pressures. Arterial pressure varies in each person depending on levels of activity and time of day. It also varies between people depending on age, elasticity of the arterial tree and the presence or absence of cardiovascular or renal disease. So a recorded systolic arterial pressure of 90 mmHg in one the individual may be low but in another may be perfectly normal.

Before deciding a patient is hypotensive, look at the preoperative check list which will indicate the preoperative pressure. Also look at the pressures recorded by the anaesthetist during the operation. These are usually lower than pre-op values. If you are in any doubt ask the anaesthetist what minimum pressure he would like maintained.

Low blood pressure may be physiological or can be induced pharmacologically by anaesthetic or sedative drugs. It can also be caused by specialized anaesthetic techniques. For instance, regional blockade such as epidural or spinal anaesthesia causes peripheral vasodilatation and consequent fall in pressure. Intermittent positive pressure ventilation reduces venous return to the right side of the heart, causing a fall in cardiac output and arterial pressure.

Hypotension may also be a pathological state due to:

- hypovalaemia (reduced blood volume)
- sepsis
- inadequate pump function of the heart (cardiogenic)
- anaphylaxis.

Hypotension due to these causes is generally termed 'shock'.

Irrespective of the causes of low pressure, if it persists it can have potentially lethal effects. The vital organs of the brain, heart and kidneys are unique in that they 'autoregulate' their blood flow. In all other tissues, blood flow will increase if arterial pressure increases and fall if the arterial pressure is low. In the vital organs, blood flow stays constant over most arterial pressures experienced by that individual. In a normotensive person, this means that the amount of blood flowing to his brain (and hence the oxygen and glucose delivered to keep the brain working) is the same whether his blood pressure is 90/40 when he is asleep or 180/90 as it may be when he is driving on a motorway. If his blood pressure falls to 60/20 during surgery, the flow of blood to his brain, heart and kidneys will fall too. As the blood pressure falls below a critical level the blood flow to these areas may diminish to the extent that insufficient oxygen and glucose reaches these areas. It is important to recognize significant hypotension, and to treat it promptly and adequately in order to avoid acute renal failure, myocardial infarction or cerebral hypoxia.

Signs and Symptoms

Arterial blood pressure is persistently at the lower end of the normal pressure range for that individual. Pressures may be expressed in terms of systolic pressure or mean pressure. If the patient is conscious they may complain of nausea, feeling light-headed or dizzy even when lying flat. They may look pale or even peripherally cyanosed (blue fingertips, earlobes or toes). They are often cold, clammy and peripherally vasoconstricted.

The arterial pressure is low whether measured invasively or non-invasively and on checking with a non-invasive sphygmomanometer. Automatic sphygmomanometers may alarm and have difficulty in measuring very low arterial pressures. It may also be difficult to get pulse oximetry readings partly because of the hypotension and partly because of peripheral vasoconstriction. If a urinary catheter is present urinary output may be poor.

Treatment

Treatment is two-pronged – supportive, ensuring adequate oxygen delivery and blood flow to vital centres, and corrective, correcting the initial pathology.

Corrective treatment depends upon the cause of the hypotension. Blood transfusion is the treatment in haemorrhagic shock, antibiotics and removal of the septic focus in septic shock, inotropic support of the heart in cardiogenic shock, and treatment of anaphylaxis in anaphylactic shock.

The mainstay of supportive treatment is to maintain oxygen delivery to the tissues until the cause of hypotension is corrected. This is achieved firstly by administering oxygen and secondly by maintaining adequate blood flow. Adequate blood flow will depend on adequate blood volume and pump function.

Oxygen must be administered at the very least by face mask but may necessitate formal intubation and artificial ventilation. Blood volume can be increased by transfusion of intravenous fluids, particularly colloids such as plasma protein substitute, or gelatin solutions but also crystalloids such as 0.9% saline or Hartmanns solution. Blood and blood products will be needed with the largest cannulae possible. Central venous cannulation can be useful both to monitor and give fluid replacement and also to give vasopressor and inotropic drugs. Pulmonary artery flotation catheters may also be introduced to measure cardiac output and monitor response to intravenous fluids and inotropes.

Pump function can be improved by adequate fluid loading and by the use of inotropic drugs. Inotropes improve the contraction of the heart, increasing the amount of blood ejected at each beat. Some inotropes have effects on the arterioles increasing the degree of vasoconstriction which will also raise the arterial pressure. All these drugs are extremely potent and are usually given diluted before being administered cautiously. Some of these drugs are given as infusions.

The anaesthetist will decide which treatment is appropriate and will give specific instructions about what is needed to his assistant.

Vasopressors

These drugs cause vasoconstriction of the arterioles and hence increase the arterial pressure. They are of particular use when the peripheral circulation is dilated and open. The patient will usually appear flushed and warm and this is most commonly seen following epidural or spinal blockade when drugs such as ephedrine or methoxamine are used. Pathological causes of vasodilatation are anaphylaxis and sepsis, when adrenaline or noradrenaline are often given.

Dopamine if infused at low rates increases renal blood flow but at higher rates of infusion also acts as a vasopressor. Dopexamine is a new agent which improves the blood flow to the kidneys and gut.

Inotropes

These drugs work by improving the contractility of the heart. Most have several other effects as well and the selection of the appropriate drug will depend upon the clinical circumstances. They are often used in conjunction with pulmonary artery flotation catheters. Examples of inotropes are adrenaline, noradrenaline, isoprenaline, dopamine, dobutamine and enoximone.

Hypertension (High Blood Pressure)

The commonest reason for an increase in blood pressure during anaesthesia is an inadequate level of anaesthesia for the surgical stimulus. This is part of the stress response to surgery. Treatment is to deepen the level of anaesthesia and/or give analgesia. Inadequate ventilation can also cause high blood pressure secondary to high CO_2 levels. In the patient with raised intracranial pressure (e.g. after a head injury) an increase in blood pressure may be secondary to a rise in intracranial pressure. Malignant hyperthemia can cause excessive CO_2 levels and hypertension. Rarely, a tumour of the adrenal gland can cause *very* high blood pressure because it secretes large amounts of adrenaline or noradrenaline.

Some patients, however, are found to have high blood pressure at the preoperative assessment and this is an important finding. Such patients are at much higher risk of suffering circulatory and cardiac problems during and after anaesthesia and surgery. If high blood pressure is untreated it can lead to heart muscle strain and damage, and damage to blood vessels (e.g. coronary arteries, renal arteries, cerebral arteries). If such a patient undergoes anaesthesia and surgery, the blood pressure can be very labile (i.e. it can plummet or shoot up) and this can lead to strokes, heart attacks and bleeding from the surgical site. So it is vitally important that high blood pressure is detected before anaesthesia and surgery and adequately controlled before the patient comes to theatre. The anaesthetist will normally have ensured this. The adequacy of blood pressure control, urgency of the surgery, drugs used to manage high blood pressure and presence of complications of high blood pressure will all affect the anaesthetic technique used. The principles of management are meticulous monitoring, ensuring careful titration of anaesthetics and analgesics and very careful postoperative care to maintain blood pressure and heart rate within the normal range and, in particular, to minimize swings up and down from the normal.

Arrhythmias (Abnormal Heart Rhythm)

Any abnormality in heart rhythm from normal sinus rhythm (but including very fast or very slow sinus rhythm) results in a fall in cardiac output. This is because the heart muscle coordination is not at its best in any other rhythm and its efficiency drops. It is important to identify abnormal rhythms before anaesthesia and surgery starts and to monitor for their occurrence during and after anaesthesia. Rhythm changes occurring during anaesthesia and their causes are listed in Table 12.1.

Table 12.1

RHYTHM	COMMON CAUSES
Slow sinus rhythm	Vagal stimulation, deep anaesthesia, too light anaesthesia, high spinal or epidural block
Fast sinus rhythm	Too light anaesthesia, stress response, atropine, ephedrine, inadequate analgesia, high CO_2, hypovolaemia, sepsis
Normal beat followed by extra beat (ectopic)	Stress response, halothane anaesthesia, high CO_2, central venous lines/wires
Very fast atrial rhythm	Stress response, coronary heart disease, atrial fibrillation, conduction disorders, hypovolaemia, sepsis
Very fast ventricular rhythm	Stress response, coronary heart disease, conduction disorders, hypoxia, sepsis, hypovolaemia
Ventricular fibrillation	Coronary heart disease, shock

SHOCK

Shock is the situation where inadequate oxygen supplies reach the tissues. It can occur because of inadequate blood flow to the tissues, inadequate oxygen in the blood or combinations of these causes. It can also occur when the tissues cannot use the oxygen, for example in cyanide poisoning. The cells need oxygen to survive and also need to be able to get rid of the waste products of metabolism, including acids and CO_2. So shock is accompanied by a build up in these acidic waste products. If not enough oxygen is supplied to cells, some can switch to a different way of deriving energy but this produces even more acid compounds and eventually the cells cannot function.

Inadequate blood flow may occur when there is a reduction in the circulating volume (hypovolaemic shock), when the heart cannot pump the blood adequately (cardiogenic shock) or in septic shock, when both mechanisms apply. In addition in septic shock, blood flow bypasses the capillary beds in the tissues as the control systems which regulate this peripheral blood flow are damaged. Thus, septic shock can be thought of as a condition in which blood flow is distributed wrongly (distributive shock).

The treatment principles are to correct low circulatory volume, optimize cardiac function and ensure correct distribution of blood flow to vital organs and peripheral tissues. Adequate oxygen supplies to the blood must be ensured and this usually means securing the airway and controlling ventilation.

13. DRUGS

N. S. Morton

ADVERSE DRUG REACTIONS

An adverse drug reaction is any drug effect that is not beneficial to the patient. Some reactions depend on the dose of drug given and are an extension of the drug's properties. This type of reaction is common, for example morphine produces dose-related depression of breathing. Other adverse reactions are not related to the dose given and are unpredictable and relatively rare, for example anaphylactic shock, malignant hyperthermia.

ANAPHYLAXIS (ANAPHYLACTIC SHOCK)

Anaphylaxis is the term used to describe an *exaggerated* response to a drug or foreign substance. This response is not related to the dose and may be caused by a tiny dose and the response is worse if exposure is repeated. The body suddenly releases large amounts of histamine and other chemicals which act on the circulatory system, the lungs and the brain. The main effects of these chemicals are to dilate the circulation and make it leaky. The patient becomes flushed and may develop patches of redness of the skin (erythema) or areas of blob-like swelling of the skin (urticaria). Itching is also common. The face, eyelids and lips may become swollen (angioedema) and, more dangerously, the airway lining may become swollen with oedema of the tissues around the larynx, posing a life-threatening situation. Because the circulation opens up suddenly and fluid leaks out rapidly into the tissues, the blood pressure falls dramatically and may lead to cardiac arrest and death as the circulation fails completely. Other effects of the released chemicals are to produce narrowing of the small airways (bronchospasm), nausea and vomiting and diarrhoea and coagulation failure with bleeding.

Triggering causes of anaphylactic shock:

- i.v. antibiotics, especially penicillins
- radiographic contrast media

- suxamethonium
- non-steroidal anti-inflammatory drugs (NSAIDs)
- some artificial colloids
- blood/blood products
- latex rubber
- peanuts and other nuts
- bee/wasp stings.

Treatment of anaphylaxis must be very prompt, as soon as it is recognized and is best thought of as a three-stage drill with

1. *immediate* treatment to ensure the airway is secure, oxygenation is adequate, bronchospasm and airway swelling reduced and low blood pressure is corrected,
2. second line treatments, and
3. further tests to identify the offending drug or foreign substance which has triggered the reaction.

The anaesthetist will give specific instructions to the assistant in this situation about how they can help.

Anaphylaxis drill (see Association of Anaesthetists guidelines – reference on page 166)

Immediate treatment

1. Stop giving the suspect drug or remove contact with the suspect foreign substance.
2. Call for help.
3. Stop the operation and anaesthesia if possible.
4. Maintain the airway and give 100% oxygen (consider tracheal intubation and ventilation).
5. Give adrenaline, intravenously 5–10 μg/kg or intraosseously (or endotracheally 100 μg/kg), give further adrenaline doses every 15 min as above if bronchospasm and hypotension persists (adrenaline produces bronchodilatation and vasoconstriction).
6. Give crystalloid/colloid 20 ml/kg rapidly.
7. Give external cardiac massage if pulse not felt or very thready.

Second line treatment

- Steroids: hydrocortisone, 4 mg/kg i.v. slowly.

- Antihistamines: chlorpheniramine, 0.2 mg/kg i.v. orally.
- Bronchodilators: salbutamol, 2.5–5 mg nebulized or 5 μg/kg slow then 1–5 μg/kg/min; i.v. aminophylline, 10 μg/kg i.v. over 1 hour, then 1.0 mg/kg/h.
- Admit to intensive care.
- Correct acidosis/hypoxaemia/hypercarbia guided by arterial blood gases and pH.
- Correct coagulation failure
- Establish invasive monitoring, arterial and CVP lines.
- Consider inotropes/vasopressors, for example noradrenaline/adrenaline.

Further tests
- Consult with immunologist and take appropriate blood tests.
- Take a careful history of other illnesses, allergies, anaesthetic problems, exposure to drugs.
- Skin prick testing after a few weeks is recommended with close supervision and full resuscitation facilities.
- Radioallergosorbent tests (RAST) can be carried out but are difficult to interpret.
- Make sure reaction is reported to the Committee on the Safety of Medicines (there are special yellow anaesthetic reaction forms for this purpose).
- Explain the problem to the patient, parent or guardian and give them a written record of the reaction.
- Encourage the patient to carry an Anaesthetic Hazard card or Medico-alert bracelet.
- Make a record in the casenotes.
- Write to the GP.

LOCAL ANAESTHETIC TOXICITY

This depends on dose, speed of injection, blood supply of the injection site, rate of clearance from the body and susceptibility to toxicity. It can thus be minimized by ensuring that a dose within safety limits is given slowly, in small divided amounts while checking by aspiration for placement of the needle in a vessel. Vasoconstrictors added to the local anaesthetic (e.g. adrenaline) reduce the maximum plasma level by reducing absorption. Care is needed to reduce doses in the neonate or where infusions are used in patients who are very ill.

If a toxic reaction occurs, it will be seen either as central nervous system symptoms (lightheadedness, ringing in the ears, numbness or tingling of the mouth and tongue, a metallic taste, visual upset, restlessness, convulsions) or as cardiovascular effects (fall in blood pressure, fall in heart rate, ventricular tachycardia). Treatment is by ensuring good oxygenation using the principles of basic and advanced life support; giving anticonvulsants (thiopentone or midazolam) and giving circulatory assistance as appropriate (cardiac massage, correction of acidosis, defibrillation, bretylium for VT, inotropes, vaso-pressors and fluids for hypotension).

SUXAMETHONIUM APNOEA

Some patients have low levels of the enzyme in their plasma which metabo-lizes suxamethonium while others have a form of the enzyme which does not work properly. This means that a normal dose of suxamethonium acts for a very long time. Breathing must be assisted until the muscle relaxation due to suxamethonium wears off and sedation or light anaesthesia must also be maintained. Blood samples should be taken to be sent for analysis of the plasma enzyme activity and the patient should be given a medic-alert card and bracelet to carry and wear. An alert should be noted prominently on the case record. Other family members may also need to be tested.

MALIGNANT HYPERTHERMIA (MH)

MH is an emergency in which the muscles unexpectedly increase their rate of metabolism. This means they use oxygen at a huge rate and produce carbon dioxide, acids, potassium and heat. As a result of this disorder the cells are flooded with calcium ions. MH is an inherited genetic disorder and can affect about 1 in 100 000 adult and 1 in 15 000 children. The gene defect has not yet been clearly identified.

MH is triggered in susceptible individuals by suxamethonium or by any of the volatile anaesthetic agents (halothane, enflurane, isoflurane, desflurane, sevoflurane). Risk factors for a MH episode are:

- previous history of MH episode
- family history of MH or anaesthetic related deaths
- abnormal muscles, especially Duchenne muscular dystrophy
- history of intolerance to caffeine
- history of fever after a previous anaesthetic.

Symptoms and signs of a MH episode are:

- increased end tidal CO_2 (an early sign)
- increased heart rate
- increase in respiratory rate
- increase in temperature (this is one reason why temperature monitoring in the theatre is so important)
- muscle stiffness
- cyanosis/desaturation
- high blood pressure
- arrhythmias.

Blood results will show:

- increase H^+ (acidosis, respiratory and metabolic)
- increase K^+ (hyperkalaemia)
- increase Mb (myoglobinaemia and myoglobinuria)
- DIC (disseminated intravascular coagulation).

Emergency treatment must be started at once. Removing the triggering agent, adequate oxygenation, active cooling and intravenous dantrolene are the most important measures. Dantrolene blocks the calcium release in the cells and so stops the cell metabolism from running in overdrive.

Emergency treatment of malignant hyperthermia (MH)

1. Stop anaesthesia and surgery.
2. Hyperventilate with 100% oxygen.
3. Give dantrolene, 2.5 mg/kg i.v.
4. Start cooling (ice packs, cold i.v. fluids, cold nasogastric, bladder irrigation or peritoneal dialysis fluid, cardiopulmonary bypass).
5. Give 1 mmol/kg sodium bicarbonate empirically and further doses as indicated by blood gas and pH measurements.
6. Establish invasive monitoring: arterial line, CVP, urinary catheter in addition to ECG, temperature, pCO_2.
7. Ensure urine output 2 ml/kg/h.
8. If all signs and symptoms have not resolved after 45 min, give dantrolene, 10 mg/kg.
9. Consider dextrose insulin for hyperkalaemia (2 ml/kg of 50% dextrose + 0.1 unit/kg insulin) (avoid calcium chloride or gluconate).

10. Consider β-blockers or procainamide for arrhythmias (avoid calcium channel blockers).

11. Continue oral/i.v. dantrolene, 1 mg/kg four times a day for 48 hours.

12. Beware later recurrence of MH (4–36 hours): continued hyperkalaemia, residual muscle rigidity, massive fluid requirements, oliguria/anuria.

DANTROLENE DOSAGE GUIDE			
DANTROLENE POWDER		**WATER**	
dantrolene sodium 20 mg ⎫			0.33 mg/ml
mannitol 3 g ⎬	+	60 ml →	dantrolene
sodium hydroxide ⎭			solution
Initial dose			
2.5 mg/kg	=	8 ml/kg	of dantrolene solution (0.33 mg/ml)
Subsequent increments			
1.0 mg/kg	=	3 ml/kg	of dantrolene solution (0.33 mg/ml)
to			
10 mg/kg	=	30 ml/kg	of dantrolene solution (0.33 mg/ml)

After the emergency is over and a few months later, the patient should have a muscle biopsy which is sent to a national testing centre in Leeds. The caffeine–halothane contracture test is used at present but it is hoped that a specific genetic test will be developed soon using DNA testing.

It is very important that the MH susceptible patient is given full information and counselling, along with their relatives. For future anaesthetics a 'trigger-free' technique is used where all the known triggering agents are avoided and an anaesthetic machine with no volatile agents leaking from black rubber components. MH susceptible patients can still have an MH episode triggered by stress and a stress-free technique with careful preoperative preparation, meticulous general anaesthesia and sedation and careful attention to postoperative pain relief are vital for success.

Patients with a definite history can be given dantrolene i.v. 2.5 mg/kg slowly over 30 min prior to induction of anaesthesia.

PORPHYRIA

This is a rare group of abnormalities of the enzyme systems in the liver which produce the oxygen carrying pigment haem (a component of

haemoglobin). An acute attack of porphyria can be triggered by some anaesthetic drugs (e.g. thiopentone). A severe attack may cause central nervous
system drainage. Safe anaesthesia involves avoiding any of the known triggering drugs, keeping the patient well hydrated, avoidance of fasting for long
periods and using known safe agents, such as propofol, morphine, bupivacaine etc.

14. EQUIPMENT

N. S. Morton

ELECTRICAL FAILURE

Most operating theatres are connected to a back up power generator electricity supply to cover the possibility of failure of the usual mains supply. This generator system is regularly checked but there is the remote chance that it could also fail. In this situation, theatre lighting, monitoring equipment and ventilators may fail. The safest option is to take over ventilation by hand using portable oxygen and a self-inflating bag and try to get a battery-powered patient monitor pack attached. The surgery should be stopped until the situation is clarified and then completed if possible as quickly as is safe. The anaesthetist will give specific instructions on how the assistant should help.

GAS SUPPLY FAILURE

The pipeline supply can fail for a variety of reasons and this is why anaesthetic machines are fitted with backup cylinders. Free-standing oxygen cylinders can also be brought into use with hand ventilation in the extreme situation of failure of all supplies from the anaesthetic machine.

FIRE

A fire in the operating theatre is an extremely dangerous event because oxygen and nitrous oxide pipeline and cylinder supplies are potentially explosive. The anaesthesia and surgery should be discontinued and the patient and personnel evacuated from the area. Oxygen supplies to the area should be isolated and cylinders removed from the area where possible. You should observe local fire drill policies and procedures and attend training in fire protection. You should familiarize yourself with fire extinguishers, fire blankets and fire exits.

Inflammable volatile anaesthetic gases are no longer used in most Western countries and so precautions against static electricity are not necessary.

INFUSION PUMP SAFETY

See Chapters 2 and 19.

ELECTROCUTION HAZARDS

There is a larger number of electrically powered pieces of equipment in modern operating theatres and these have to be checked and certified for electrical safety by the hospital physicist or bioengineer. You should only use equipment according to manufacturer's instructions and avoid fluid spillages onto electrical equipment. If a fault is noted, the equipment must be taken out of service until repaired professionally. Do not attempt do-it-yourself work!

DIATHERMY

Where surgical diathermy is to be used, you should ensure the patient plate electrode is correctly applied to a smooth flat surface, is of the correct size and is connected correctly to the machine. It is good practise to ask a colleague to double check this.

15. FLUIDS

N. S. Morton

TRANSFUSION REACTIONS

The commonest cause of blood transfusion reactions is failure to check blood correctly with a double check by another member of staff. Only doctors and nurses should check blood.

Blood transfusion reactions may present in a variety of ways. The commonest early signs are fever, shivering, rashes or anaphylaxis. Later signs include jaundice and anaemia due to red cell breakdown.

The treatment on suspicion of a transfusion reaction is firstly to stop the transfusion, disconnect the blood-giving set from the patient and save the unit of blood for further testing. Oxygen should be given and anaphylaxis drill may have to be started. Further patient blood samples may be needed to work out the reason for the reaction. The assistant will be given specific instructions by the anaesthetist in this situation.

MASSIVE TRANSFUSION

Rapid transfusion of large amounts of intravenous fluids, colloids, blood or blood products can cause problems of dilution of coagulation factors, damage to the lungs due to deposition of clumps of debris and cells from transfused blood, and a sudden fall in the level of calcium in the patient's blood. This latter effect is significant in small babies who are receiving rapid infusion of fresh frozen plasma or blood as the citrate anticoagulant from the administered packs tend to bind the patient's calcium. In neonates, this can cause a deterioration in cardiac function and so calcium replacement is given.

It is debatable whether filters incorporated into infusion sets are necessary and a balance needs to be struck in each case between the need to transfuse quickly and the inevitable slowing of the infusion rate when a filter is used. There is some evidence that forcing stored blood through filters damages the cellular elements in the transfused blood so in many centres filters are no longer used.

The lung damage due to massive transfusion is a form of pulmonary oedema or adult respiratory distress syndrome (ARDS) where excessive fluid leaks into the gas-exchanging parts of the lung and into the interstitial space in the lung. The effect is to make the lungs waterlogged and stiff, and to impede gas exchange.

It is hard to prevent these effects of massive transfusion, but they may influence treatment that has to be given to the patient in the theatre and thereafter, for example regular checks and correction of coagulation parameters, blood gases and ventilator settings.

KEY LEARNING POINTS

- Be prepared for emergencies at all times before, during and after anaesthesia.

- Ensure you know where resuscitation drugs and equipment are located

- Ensure you know by heart the protocols for basic and advanced life support for adults and children

Further Reading

'Guidelines for basic life support', European Resuscitation Council. Resuscitation 1992; 24: 103–110.
'Guidelines for advanced life support', European Resuscitation Council. Resuscitation 1992; 24L 111–121.
'Guidelines for paediatric life support', European Resuscitation Council. Resuscitation 1992; 27: 91–105.
'Advanced Paediatric Life support', Advanced Life Support Group. BMJ Publishing Group, London, 1993.
'Anaphylactic reactions associated with anaesthesia', Association of Anaesthetists, London, 1990.
'Intensive Care: A Concise Textbook', 2nd edition. CJ Hind, D Watson, WB Saunders, London, 1996.
'Paediatric Intensive Care'. NS Morton, Oxford Medical Publications, Oxford, 1997.

Relevance

ODP Level 3   Units 6, 7, 8.

SECTION 5

RECOVERY AND POSTOPERATIVE CARE

16. EQUIPPING AND STAFFING THE RECOVERY AREA

E. Holmes, N. S. Morton

It is now expected that all patients after surgery will be cared for in a designated recovery area. Many hospitals have such an area adjacent to or integrated into the operating theatre suite while others have had to reorganize space or improvise from smaller spaces. A recovery room is a specialist area providing specific individualized care for all postoperative patients with a high ratio of trained nursing staff to patients. This is vital for patient safety as up to 1 in 5 of all complications after surgery and anaesthesia occur in the early postoperative period. Some recovery areas also act in part as high dependency units for patients who need closer observation than can be provided in the general ward but who do not need intensive care. The staffing of such a high dependency area must be more intense.

The criteria for admission to the recovery area include patients who are recovering from procedures under general anaesthesia, sedation or regional anaesthesia. A reception area is usually set aside for patients before their surgery. This area must be adequately staffed to undertake the handover of care from the ward staff, to look after patients who have had sedative premedication and to reassure patients who may be anxious while waiting. If children are also received into this area, a section should be set aside for them separate from adults, with child-safe and friendly surroundings. Qualified paediatric nurses are necessary wherever children are looked after.

In some reception areas the patient receives premedication upon arrival and other preparations for anaesthesia and surgery can also be carried out here. For example, regional blocks can be carried out in reception with appropriate safeguards and this can improve the operating theatre throughput.

The recovery area staff should have good lines of communication to laboratories, radiology, pharmacy, portering, patient transfer and the resuscitation team. Clerical staff can be employed to answer telephones, relay messages and undertake secretarial duties and this is helpful in freeing nursing staff for direct patient care.

Recovery Area Space

Large open rooms are easier to manage as all patients can be seen and heard, staff can communicate quickly and work flexibly to help each other when the unit is busy. However, they can be difficult to heat and ventilate and privacy for patients can be a problem. Natural light is preferable and the temperature of the room needs to be at least 23°C to reduce postoperative heat loss and shivering. The large area can be partitioned using moveable screens, work stations or curtains. Specific treatment areas for patients who require ventilatory support, regional blocks, X-rays, more intensive monitoring, isolation because of infection or radium implants, or an area for children can all be delineated.

Each patient must have his own bed or trolley with plenty of room for the staff to work around the patient and have easy access to the necessary equipment and services. Incorporated into each patient space must be an oxygen supply, suction equipment and electrical points. Monitoring equipment and work surfaces may be mobile or fixed at each space. It is important that this area should not be shared with another patient in case an emergency arises.

There must be adequate storage space for monitoring equipment, drugs, emergency equipment, intravenous equipment and fluids, medical gas cylinders, sterile supplies, linen, trolleys, beds, lifting and traction equipment. There must be a disposal room for soiled linen, dressings and toilet articles.

Recovery Area Equipment

It is essential that each bed space has its own supply of equipment stored in a mobile unit, drawers or on shelves or worktops.

Essential items at each bed space are:

- oxygen supply, tubing, masks, T-piece connections for laryngeal mask airway, nasal cannulae, nebulisers, orophryngeal airways, nasopharyngeal airways
- suction unit, tubing, soft suction catheters, rigid (Yankauer) suction tubes
- ECG monitor, leads, electrodes, pressure transducers
- pulse oximeter
- non-invasive blood pressure cuffs
- thermometers
- i.v. cannulae, needles, syringes, skin prep swabs, adhesive tape, dressings
- disposable gloves

- tissues, disposal bags, sharps box, vomit bowls
- relevant charts.

Essential items immediately accessible in the recovery area are:
- resuscitation equipment
- self-inflating bags
- anaesthetic machine
- ventilator
- intubation equipment and aids
- difficult intubation kit
- mobile oxygen cylinder and flowmeter
- mobile suction unit
- peripheral and central vascular access equipment
- chest drains and underwater seal kits
- intravenous fluids
- nerve stimulator
- blood sample tubes, blood culture bottles
- blood glucose monitor
- bladder catheters, urinometers, irrigation systems and fluids, urine testing kits
- warming equipment for patient (warm air, electric, water, foil), i.v. fluids
- cooling equipment (fans, ice packs)
- linen, dressings, drains, drainage bags
- lifting and moving aids.

Drugs which should be immediately available are:
- analgesics
- antibiotics
- anticholinergics
- antiemetics
- antihistamines
- antihypertensives
- antiarrhythmics
- steroids
- inotropes
- diuretics
- resuscitation drugs
- muscle relaxants
- reversal agents for relaxants, opioids, benzodiazepines
- local anaesthetics.

Each recovery unit has its own policy in relation to the checking and stocking of equipment with a minimum of a documented daily check by a responsible nurse. Any faults in equipment or gaps in the stock of equipment, drugs or fluids should be corrected as soon as possible.

RECOVERY AREA STAFFING

The staffing levels in the recovery area depend on the case load, case mix and turnover of cases on the operating lists. Staff should be appropriately trained and the unit will function best with a variety of grades of personnel. The skill mix should be balanced with a senior nurse carrying overall responsibility for the management of the unit, for patient care and for staff. There should be an active teaching and audit program in the unit but releasing staff to attend teaching sessions can be difficult. Certain skills need to be regularly re-tested, for example resuscitation. Training and assessment of competence should be undertaken according to nationally recognized standards. It is useful if staff employed in recovery areas have experience of working in an acute care setting such as an intensive care unit, an acute receiving unit or operating theatre as the skills gained in these areas are those essential for recovery staff.

Some large hospitals have an anaesthetist resident whose sole duties are to manage patients in the recovery area. This is very helpful in providing immediate resuscitation, monitoring and analgesia skills and in coordinating the input from the various specialities such as surgery, radiology, anaesthesia and nursing.

RECOVERY AREA PROTOCOLS, POLICIES AND GUIDELINES

It is essential that local unit policies are drawn up regarding emergencies, resuscitation, drug administration, infectious cases, radiation protection, accidents, admission criteria and discharge criteria.

17. Monitoring the Recovering Patient

E. Holmes, N. S. Morton

The main aim of recovery care is to ensure the patient's safety and comfort in the early postoperative period and has been defined as protective care. This is complimentary to the principles of 'total' safety of the patient in the operating department.

Coordination of care amongst the different specialty groups, good communication, clear documentation and a plan of care are helpful safety features.

Transfer of the patient from theatre to recovery is usually carried out by the patient's anaesthetist, the anaesthetic assistant and/or a theatre nurse. In some units the recovery staff collect the patient from the anaesthetist in a handover area in theatre. The transfer arrangements will depend on the layout and design of the operating theatres and recovery facilities.

The nurse who accepts the patient must know the details of the patient in advance and be told about the procedure in theatre and about any problems during surgery or anticipated in the early postoperative phrase. Make sure that the patient is correctly positioned on the trolly or bed, that the airway is maintained and the patient is stable from the respiratory and cardivascular points of view. They must know how to tip the trolley or bed head down, know how the braking mechanism on the trolley works and that the bed sides are up so that the patient cannot roll off. The unconscious patient must never be left unattended and must have at least one-to-one nursing care.

A to F of Recovery

An alphabetical scheme will help you to assess the recovering patient:

- airway
- breathing
- circulation
- conscious level
- drains, dressings, drugs

- elimination
- fluid balance.

Informed clinical observation is the most efficient way to monitor, identify and treat important problems during the recovery period. The priority is to ensure patency of the airway at all times. It is advisable to nurse the patient on their side in the recovery position which helps maintain the airway and prevents the tongue falling back to cause airway obstruction in the extubated patient. Secretions, blood, regurgitated stomach contents and vomit will pool in the mouth or come out onto the bed rather than being aspirated into the lungs. Chin lift and jaw thrust manoeuvres may be required to support the patient's airway until they are conscious enough to maintain their own airway. In some cases, it may not be possible to have the patient on his side because of the type of surgery, for example spinal surgery, hip replacement surgery. In such cases meticulous control of the airway is essential until the patient recovers consciousness. Secretions, blood or vomit should be removed by suctioning. An oropharyngeal or nasopharyngeal airway may help to maintain the airway but occasionally some patients may require reintubation to establish and secure the airway, for example those with laryngeal spasm or laryngeal oedema. Partially obstructed breathing is noisy with see-sawing movements of the chest and abdomen. The patient who has these movements but no breath sounds has complete airway obstruction. Ensure the patient is receiving high flow oxygen, at least 40%, and check that the skin, nail beds and mucous membranes of the lips and tongue are pink and that the pulse oximetry values are >94%. Is the breathing rate normal, very fast, very slow or zero? If anything other than normal you must immediately bring this to the attention of the anaesthetist, support the airway, give oxygen and commence bag and mask ventilation if the patient is not breathing. Residual effects of the anaesthetic drugs, muscle relaxants and especially opioids can cause slowing or arrest of breathing and remember that apnoea can be a complication of high central local anaesthetic blocks (e.g. a total spinal). Remember there are specific antagonists for opioids (naloxone) and benzodiazepines (flumazenil) and some agents can stimulate the breathing centre in the brain (doxapram).

Oxygen delivery to the tissues depends on adequate supplies of oxygen reaching the blood, adequate cardiac output and correct distribution of that cardiac output to the tissues. Hypoxia due to airway obstruction or inadequate breathing can cause circulatory problems. Slowing of the heart rate, asystole and abnormal rhythms such as ventricular ectopics, ventricular tachycardia and ventricular fibrillation can all occur. The hypoxia must be corrected first and specific antiarrhythmic drugs may be needed. In children, slowing of the heart rate is nearly always due to hypoxia and diagnosis and intervention to open the airway, give extra oxygen an assist ventilation must be immediate.

If the pulse is absent then full CPR procedures must be started at once. Abnormal heart rate or rhythm should be drawn to the attention of the anaesthetist at once as it may be pre-existing, due to drugs, or secondary to respiratory, neurological, cardiac or surgical problems.

The adequacy of blood flow to the tissues can be judged from the combination of blood pressure, heart rate, skin colour, skin temperature, capillary refill time and urine output. A low cardiac output will cause a fall in SpO_2.

Conscious level can be assessed using Guedel's stages of anaesthesia and this has the advantage of checking for return of protective airway reflexes. Another useful simple assessment of conscious level is the AVPU scheme:

- Awake
- responds to Verbal stimuli
- responds to Painful stimuli
- Unresponsive.

This can be qualified by assessing whether the response is appropriate or not.

The aim is to have the patient awake or gently asleep and responding appropriately to spoken commands.

The site and type of drains must be documented and losses charted accurately. Excessive losses must be drawn to the attention of the anaesthetist and specialist drains such as underwater seal systems must be checked to ensure they are set up correctly and continue to function properly.

Drugs given in theatre should be noted and any to be given in the recovery area must be correctly prescribed and administered by suitably qualified and certified staff. Some staff are able to give i.v. drugs and change infusion fluids and equipment. Analgesics, local anaesthetics and antiemetics are the commonest drugs given in recovery (see Chapter 19).

Fluid balance must be carefully maintained according to instructions from the anaesthetist and surgeon and this will involve accurate recording of fluid inputs and outputs. Drain losses, nasogastric drainage and urine output need to be measured regularly and excessive losses or inadequate urine output drawn to the anaesthetists attention.

A CHECKLIST FOR RECOVERY

- airway
- breathing
- circulation
- conscious level
- drains, dressings, drugs
- elimination
- fluids
- notes, records, charts, X-rays
- temperature monitoring and maintenance
- positioning
- pain control
- control of postoperative nausea and vomiting
- hygiene
- fitness for discharge assessment
- handover to ward.

18. DIAGNOSIS AND MANAGEMENT OF EARLY POSTOPERATIVE PROBLEMS

E. Holmes, G. Gillies

RESPIRATORY PROBLEMS

An early feature of most respiratory problems when the patient is breathing room air is a fall in oxygen saturation revealed by the pulse oximeter. This can be treated by administering oxygen whilst further help is summoned. If the patient is apnoeic or is making very little respiratory effort, positive pressure ventilation by self-inflating bag and mask should be given by the assistant or anaesthetist or a tracheal tube should be inserted by the anaesthetist without delay.

Airway Obstruction

The classic signs of airway obstruction are see-saw paradoxical movements of chest and abdomen and noisy stridorous breathing noises, although there will be no breath sounds if airway obstruction is complete. Common causes are the tongue, foreign body or debris, blocked, kinked or misplaced artificial airway (oropharyngeal, LMA, tracheal tube) and laryngospasm. Laryngeal oedema can occur as a local reaction (e.g. latex allergy) or as part of an anaphylactoid response. In children mucosal oedema at the level of the cricoid ring can occur after extubation due to the use of too large an endotracheal tube.

Hypoventilation with Central Depression

Depression of the respiratory centre occurs with any sedative agent but is seen most commonly in association with opioids. The patient may be apnoeic or exhibit the characteristic breathing pattern of deep, sighing respirations with a low respiratory rate. The pupils are pin-point and the patient may respond to prompting to breathe but will lapse when unstimulated or may be unrousable. There is a wide variation between individuals in their response to opioids, with the neonate and the elderly particularly sensitive to their effects.

If respiration is inadequate, positive pressure ventilation must be commenced until the patient's respiratory drive is adequate.

Doxapram, up to 1.0 mg/kg, is a centrally acting respiratory stimulant which increases respiratory rate and depth and is often associated with a lightening of conscious level. It can be given as small intravenous increments or as a continuous infusion. It can cause excitatory side-effects such as restlessness and convulsions and can cause high blood pressure.

Naloxone, 10 µg/kg, is a specific opioid antagonist which rapidly reverses opioid-induced sedation, respiratory depression and, unfortunately, analgesia. This latter effect means that patients may become very distressed and restless due to pain after naloxone is given. The effects of naloxone are quite short lived and there is a risk of resedation as the effects wear off especially if large doses of opioids have been given. Repeated doses of 10 µg/kg can be given or a continuous infusion of 10 µg/kg/h may be used. Alternatively, a larger dose (100 µg/kg) can be given i.m.

For benzodiazepine-induced sedation the specific antagonist flumazenil, 5 µg/kg, can be given and may have to be repeated because of its relatively short duration of effect, up to a total dose of 40 µg/kg.

Residual Paralysis, Incomplete Reversal of Muscle Relaxants, Recurarization

This is seen less commonly since the introduction of shorter acting muscle relaxants and the more widespread use of peripheral nerve simulators. Incomplete reversal of non-depolarizing muscle relaxants is most likely to occur in association with a relative overdose, especially in the neonate or the elderly. Reversal may also be affected by acidosis (e.g. in shock or respiratory failure), low potassium, hypothermia and drug interactions (e.g. aminoglycoside antibiotics such as gentamicin). Patients with muscle diseases such as myasthenia gravis are sensitive to muscle relaxant drugs.

Two muscle relaxant drugs in common use are broken down by an enzyme in the blood, namely serum cholinesterase. These are the depolarizing relaxant suxamethonium and the non-depolarizing relaxant mivacurium. Some patients have low levels of activity of this enzyme due to a genetic abnormality and this leads to a standard dose having a very prolonged effect (i.e. hours instead of minutes).

Patients recovering from anaesthesia with incomplete reversal of neuromuscular block may be apnoeic or have reduced respiratory excursions. Respiratory efforts may be associated with jerky movements of the diaphragm and gasping respirations with a tracheal tug (jerky movements of the thyroid cartilage on inspiration). Limb movements, if any, are spasmodic and uncoordinated. The patient has a weak cough. If consciousness has returned, the patient may be distressed with an associated tachycardia and hypertension. The diagnosis can be confirmed using a peripheral nerve stimulator which will show absence or fade of the train-of-four (TOF) response.

Treatment depends on correcting the underlying cause, giving oxygen and ventilatory support and considering giving a second dose of reversal agent.

Hypocapnic Apnoea (Low CO_2 Stores)

Any patient who has been overventilated will have low CO_2 stores and a low arterial pCO_2. As the respiratory centre is stimulated by CO_2, a low level will tend to lead to a period of underventilation or apnoea. Patients who have had opioids are even more likely to show this effect.

Reflex Laryngeal Apnoea

Patients lightening from anaesthesia with an endotracheal tube in place may breath hold as a reflex response to stimulation of the larynx and trachea by the tube. It is more common in patients with respiratory disease, respiratory infections and in smokers.

Diffusion Hypoxia

If the patient has been anaesthetized with a mixture containing nitrous oxide, the lungs and tissues will have accumulated a lot of nitrous oxide. If the patient is allowed to breathe room air (21% oxygen) immediately after surgery, the nitrous oxide diffuses out very rapidly and dilutes the oxygen in the airways and gas exchanging sacs in the lungs. This leads to a reduction in the oxygen available to be taken up into the circulation from the lungs and arterial oxygen levels can fall to critically low levels. This effect can be prevented by giving patients oxygen to breathe at the end of surgery until the nitrous oxide has been washed out. In young fit patients this may not take very long but in the elderly or in those with significant lung disease it can take hours.

Pneumothorax

The presence of air within the pleural space (outside the lung but within the thorax) is referred to as a pneumothorax. It can occur whenever there is a hole in the pleural membrane covering the lung or the thoracic cavity communicates with the air. The lung tends to collapse and sometimes the pocket of air can expand and become pressurized (a tension pneumothorax). The heart and trachea can be pushed over to the opposite side and the filling of the heart can be reduced by compression of the great veins and heart chambers.

The patient with a pneumothorax may complain of a sharp chest pain on the affected side when breathing in or may have difficulty in breathing (dyspnoea) or develop rapid shallow breathing (tachypnoea). The chest expansion on the side of the pneumothorax may be less and the breath sounds on that side will be reduced. The chest may sound hyperresonant on percussion on the side of the pneumothorax. A chest X-ray will confirm the diagnosis but if the pneumo-thorax is under tension a needle should be inserted into the thoracic cavity to release the air without waiting for an X-ray. A chest drain should then be inserted under local anaesthesia and connected to an underwater seal system.

A pneumothorax can occur spontaneously, but is usually associated with trauma, lung biopsies, CVP line insertions, intercostal blocks, supraclavicular brachial plexus blocks, chest surgery, cardiac surgery and kidney surgery.

Pulmonary Oedema

This occurs most commonly in patients with poor cardiac function who have had more fluid than their heart can cope with. It is also a feature of septic shock, chest trauma, smoke inhalation, aspiration of gastric contents and massive transfusion of blood or blood products.

Patients may be distressed and exhibit dyspnoea and tachypnoea with a tachycardia. Their breathing may be audibly moist and there may be a productive cough with pink or white frothy sputum. Oxygen, diuretics, fluid restriction and inotropic support may all be needed.

Mechanical and Positional Effects on Respiratory Function

After abdominal surgery, air in the peritoneum and bowel distension causes splinting of the diaphragm and wound pain tends to make the patient take shallow breaths. Lying down also restricts breathing, especially in the obese patient. Areas of lung tend to be underventilated and tend to collapse down (atelectasis) and these areas do not take part in gas exchange. This causes a fall in arterial oxygenation (intrapulmonary shunting). The sitting position helps and additional inspired oxygen will help correct the low arterial oxygen levels. Good pain relief and physiotherapy are essential.

Acute Bronchospasm

This is caused by narrowing of the small airways and is associated with breathlessness and wheeze mainly during expiration. It occurs most commonly in patients with asthma or chronic obstructive airways disease. It may occur in response to laryngeal or tracheal irritation, as a drug side effect (e.g. beta blockers or NSAIDs) or as part of an anaphylactoid response. Treatment involves administration of oxygen and i.v. or nebulized bronchodilators. Aminophylline or salbutamol are the most-often used.

Acid Aspiration Syndrome

This is where upper gastrointestinal contents or food pass into the lungs and can occur at induction, during the anaesthetic or during recovery. A drop in oxygen saturation which does not readily respond to oxygen or increased ventilatory support may be seen. Bronchospasm, dyspnoea, tachypnoea, pulmonary oedema and hypoxia are seen and the chest X-ray will show infiltrates and areas of collapse and consolidation. Immediate treatment includes tracheal intubation, suctioning of the trachea and main airways, ventilatory support, bronchodilators, steroids and antibiotics.

High Local Anaesthetic Block

Epidural and spinal anaesthesia can result in respiratory difficulty if the block comes too high and involves the intercostal muscles and the nerves supplying the diaphragm. The epidural catheter could puncture the dura and if the usual top-up dose is given inadvertently into the subarachnoid space a high or total spinal block will result. This can also occur as a complication of other blocks such as paravertebral blocks or retrobullar blocks.

At Risk Patients

After abdominal and thoracic surgery there may be persistent problems with gas exchange for the reasons noted above and patients may need supplemental oxygen, analgesia and physiotherapy for 3–7 days. Patients with previous respiratory and cardiac disease are at high risk of breathing problems after surgery.

CIRCULATORY PROBLEMS

If blood or other fluid losses are not adequately replaced then CVP, arterial pressure and urine output tend to be low, with an increase in heart rate. In some patients with major blood loss the syndrome of DIC occurs (disseminated intravascular coagulation). Clots forming throughout the circulation consumes clotting factors and this means that any wounds or puncture sites tend to ooze and bleed. Blood tests of the clotting mechanism are used to identify specific clotting defects and coagulation factors can be replaced. Transfusions of fresh frozen plasma, platelets and cryoprecipitate are most commonly used for this purpose.

HYPOTHERMIA

Heat loss during surgery is common and is especially likely in babies (see Chapter 30), and during major or prolonged surgery. Heat is lost via the airway, from exposure of body surfaces and body cavities by radiation to surroundings and by evaporative losses especially from the lungs and open body cavities.

Anaesthetic gases are dry and cold and the patient has to try to humidify and heat the gases via the airway lining. If a high fresh gas flow is used for a long time, then considerable heat can be lost. Heat and humidity can be conserved using circle systems with carbon dioxide absorbers and low fresh gas flows. Another option is to use a heat and moisture exchanger in the breathing circuit.

For body cavity losses, warm packs, warm irrigating fluids, minimizing exposure and short operating times are helpful. For body surface losses, covering exposed areas with foil, plastic, gamgee or drapes is helpful. Active warming using water mattresses, electric blankets or warm air systems is useful in theatre and recovery. Warming intravenous fluids can now be carried out efficiently using coil warming systems which have thermostatic control. Old-style water bath systems are useless and dangerous because of the electrocution hazard.

Hypothermia tends to cause the peripheral circulation to shut down, which puts an extra load on the heart and impairs perfusion of the tissues. On rewarming this circulation opens up and the arterial pressure tends to fall. Acid waste products are washed out of the tissues and this can impair heart function and puts an extra load on the respiratory system. Shivering in response to a fall in body temperature leads to consumption of extra oxygen and thus oxygen supplies must be increased to cope with this extra demand. Any shivering patient must be given extra oxygen until they are fully rewarmed.

Hyperthermia

Pyrexia after surgery may be related to a fever before surgery (especially in emergency intrabdominal cases), due to bacteraemia or septicaemia induced during surgery (e.g. urology), due to chest infections or more rarely due to malignant hyperthermia. Specimens for culture and blood cultures may be needed and antibiotics given. Pyrexia is common in the first 24 hours after surgery as a response to tissue injury but chest complications and deep venous thrombosis are common causes of postoperative fever.

19. PREVENTION AND CONTROL OF PAIN

N. S. Morton

In modern practice, pain should be anticipated and pain killers given before the tissues are injured, whenever possible. There are good reasons for this. It is now known that by giving pain relief before the painful wound occurs, less pain-producing substances are released by the wounded tissues and the area near to the wound is less sensitive in the period after the operation. The non-steroidal anti-inflammatory drugs (NSAIDs) such as aspirin, ibuprofen, diclofenac and ketorolac produce most of their pain-killing effect by working in this way in the tissues. If less pain-producing substances are in or near the wound, fewer pain signals will pass along the nerve fibres to the spinal cord and on to the brain. These signals can be further blocked during their passage along the nerves by the use of local anaesthetic agents applied near to the nerves themselves or near to the spinal cord (subarachnoid block, epidural block). Opioids such as morphine, diamorphine or fentanyl can be given near to the spinal cord and act locally on opioid receptors in the spinal cord to block pain signals. Opioids also act in the brain to reduce pain by acting upon opioid receptors and by causing some degree of sedation. General anaesthesia with gaseous and/or intravenous anaesthetics reduces the patient's ability to feel pain by depressing consciousness. Painful signals can however still reach the brain and cause adverse effects unless very deep levels of anaesthesia are used. Thus, many anaesthetists now use combinations of these pain-relieving techniques given before the painful stimulus takes place to try to block several different parts of the pain pathway at once (Fig 19.1). After surgery, analgesia can be continued safely for as long as required provided patients are nursed and monitored appropriately. This is best done in the context of a properly organized pain relief service (Tables 19.1; 19.2). There is a lot of merit in trained anaesthetic assistants becoming involved in the pain relief service.

Modern pain prevention relies upon good local or regional analgesia, safe use of opioids and adequate doses of concurrently administered NSAIDs or paracetamol. Sedation or general anaesthesia also contribute to optimum pain prevention. This three-pronged attack on the pain pathways is often called

- **TISSUES**
  local anaesthetics eg. EMLA cream, amethocaine gel, lignocaine gel
  NSAIDs eg. aspirin, ibuprofen, diclofenac, ketorolac

- **PERIPHERAL NERVES**
  local anaesthetics eg. peripheral nerve block

- **SPINAL CORD**
  local anaesthetics eg. epidural or subarachnoid block
  opioids

- **BRAIN**
  general anaesthetics
  nitrous oxide
  opioids
  paracetamol

Fig. 19.1 Sites of action of drugs used to block the main pathways

Table 19.1

ACUTE PAIN RELIEF SERVICE	
ROLES	**METHODS**
organisation	multidisciplinary team (anaesthesia, surgery, pharmacy, nursing, physiotherapy, medical specialties)
provision	ward rounds, follow-up visits
education	teaching ward rounds, lectures, tutorials, distance learning
audit	monitoring, data collection, incident reporting
research	evaluation of techniques, comparative studies

'balanced analgesia'. The fact that the analgesia is started before the surgical stimulus where possible is known as 'pre-emptive analgesia'.

TECHNIQUES OF PAIN PREVENTION AND PAIN RELIEF

Local Anaesthetic Techniques

The commonly used techniques were described in Chapter 4. Most rely on a single dose of a long acting local anaesthetic such as bupivacaine to produce

Table 19.2

COMMON PAIN RELIEVING DRUGS AND THEIR DOSES				
DRUG	**DOSAGE**	**ROUTE**	**SITES OF ACTION**	**USES**
paracetamol	10–20 mg/kg, q4–6 h	o,r	tissues, brain	mild pain/adjunct
NSAIDS (not in child < age 1y)				
ibuprofen	2.5–10 mg/kg, q6 h	o	tissues	mod pain/adjunct
diclofenac	1–1.5 mg/kg, q8 h	o,r	tissues	mod pain/adjunct
ketorolac	0.1–0.3 mg/kg, q6 h	iv,im	tissues	mod pain/adjunct
OPIOIDS				
codeine	0.5–1 mg/kg	o,im	brain	mod pain
dihydrocodeine	0.5–1 mg/kg	o,im	brain	mod pain
tramadol	1–2 mg/kg	o,im,iv	brain	mod/severe pain
morphine	0.1–0.2 mg/kg	o,im,iv,sc	brain	severe pain
	5–30 mcg/kg/h	infusion	brain	severe pain

several hours of postoperative local or regional analgesia. Some techniques can be repeated, for example intercostal nerve blocks, but most patients find this unpleasant. Another option is to place an indwelling cannula or catheter in the nerve plexus sheath or in the epidural space. Top-ups of bupivacaine can be given when required or an infusion of bupivacaine can be run with supplementary top-ups if required. The advantage of infusions is that the number of top-ups is much reduced which is more efficient in terms of the anaesthetist's time. In some centres, nursing staff and midwives are trained to administer local anaesthetic top-ups and adjust infusions.

These patients need a high dependency level of nursing care and some will need intensive care. There is still controversy about whether such patients can be looked after in general wards, but many centres are doing so. However, they have to ensure that the level of monitoring is adequate and that anaesthetic help is readily available to deal with problems.

Many centres add opioids to the epidural bupivacaine solutions, for example fentanyl, diamorphine, sufentanil, morphine. The safety of such methods is currently being evaluated as the epidural opioids can cause ventilatory depression, sedation, nausea and vomiting, itching and urinary retention.

In children, epidurals can be used provided doses are adjusted. These techniques can be applied to neonates, infants and older children if correct procedures are followed.

Opioid Techniques

Opioids are drugs related to morphine and they act on opioid receptors in the brain and spinal cord to produce pain relief (analgesia). The commonly used opioids and their properties are shown in Table 19.2.

The 'gold standard' is still morphine and it is the most commonly used opioid. Morphine can be administered by a variety of routes but it is most often given by injection. The traditional intramuscular (i.m.) injection of morphine prescribed 'as required' is not very satisfactory because many patients are reluctant to disturb staff to ask for an injection and many patients (especially children) do not like injections. From the nursing staff's view-point, i.m. injections are time consuming to draw up, check and administer because the Controlled Drug regulations demand that two qualified staff should perform this task. After an i.m. injection of morphine the drug is absorbed relatively slowly into the bloodstream but reaches quite a high peak level and then declines over the next 2 or 3 hours. This means that pain relief is slow to come on, lasts a relatively short time and, when the peak blood levels of morphine are circulating, there are more side-effects. The net result is a saw tooth pattern of severe pain, injection, side-effects and short-lived analgesia (Figs 19.2 & 19.3).

This situation can be improved by a protocol for giving i.m. morphine and this does result in more effective analgesia. The key principles for the safe use

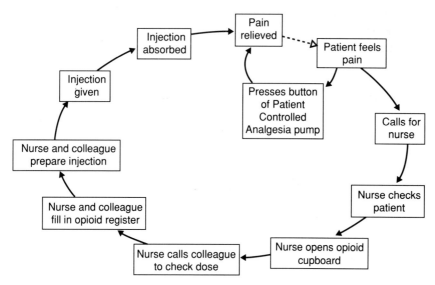

Fig. 19.2 The long circuit for intramuscular analgesia contrasts with the short circuit for patient-controlled analgesia

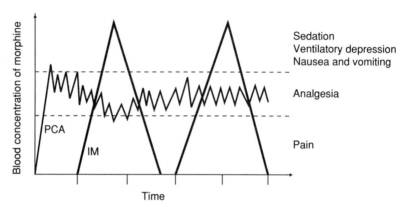

Fig. 19.3 Intermittent intramuscular injections cause swings in blood concentration with periods of no analgesia or adverse effects. PCA allows the patient to titrate their pain relief to achieve acceptable analgesia with minimal side effects

of opioids are to *titrate* the dose carefully to each patient's response and to reassess regularly the level of pain and the occurrence and severity of adverse effects. This does not require a huge input of new resources but simply good nursing and medical observation while individualizing care to allow for the huge variation between patients in their need for analgesia.

Another approach to i.m. morphine administration is to place an i.m. cannula through which top-up doses of morphine or a continuous infusion can be given. This avoids repeated needle sticks and is used in some paediatric centres.

Morphine can also be given under the skin (subcutaneous; s.c.) by intermittent injection or through an indwelling cannula. These injections behave just like i.m. injections. With both i.m. and s.c. morphine, care is needed in the patient who has a poor circulation to the skin or muscle. In the postoperative period, particularly after major surgery, fluid shifts and cold may result in a decrease in the circulation to the muscles and skin which then improves later with rewarming and fluid therapy. This can result in a 'wash out' of morphine from the i.m. or s.c. sites into the circulation, which then produces respiratory depression.

Subcutaneous infusion of morphine is particularly useful in children because it can be used in any age of child, does not rely on keeping a small peripheral vein open (which can be particularly difficult in small babies), is easy to secure and is very well tolerated. Safety aspects must be meticulous. The warning about ensuring that the peripheral circulation is adequate and stable is equally important in children. A s.c. cannula can be placed while the child is anaesthetized or under EMLA cream cover. The best sites are on the upper arm over the outer aspect of the deltoid region, over the lower anterior abdominal wall or over the outer aspect of the thigh. A spiral type of extension line between the pump and the patient is very helpful in allowing the child some mobility.

The s.c. route was the original way for giving Patient-Controlled Analgesia (PCA) described in the 1960s. The patient called the nurse when in pain and was given a s.c. bolus of morphine. With the development of infusion pumps, special patient-activated pumps were designed. These have become more sophisticated so that a wide range of dosage protocols can be used and matched to each patient. The cost of these pumps is quite high so non-electronic PCA devices have been developed which work perfectly well but lack the flexibility of electronic devices.

The principle of PCA is based on the idea that the best judge of their pain is the patient. They are given access to pain relief via the prescription programmed into the PCA device by the anaesthetist. This prescription describes the analgesic drug (usually morphine), the volume of drug in the syringe and its concentration. The dose delivered with each patient demand is determined by the anaesthetist and the time interval before the patient gets another dose is also set at between 5 and 10 minutes. This interval is called the lockout time as the patient can make demands during this time but will not have a dose delivered by the pump. The logic behind a lockout time is to allow a period after each bolus of morphine for the effect to reach its peak which usually takes up to 10 minutes in most patients. If there was no lockout time, it would be possible for the patient to make rapidly repeated demands one after the other which would accumulate into a large dose with resulting side-effects. So the lockout time allows the patient to feel almost the full effect of a single demand bolus dose and decide for him/herself if it is giving adequate pain relief. If not, they simply make another demand. Over a short time the patient learns to self-titrate to an acceptable level of comfort. Morphine does produce adverse effects (Table 19.3) and some patients using PCA morphine limit their demands because of effects such as nausea and vomiting. So, as well as self-titrating to acceptable analgesia, the patient also self-titrates to an acceptable level of side-effects. The pump settings may have to be adjusted to allow optimum analgesia to be achieved for each individual. This is best done by frequently reassessing and monitoring pain and adverse effects.

Another aspect of the PCA prescription which can be varied is the ability to run a continuous infusion of morphine in the background while the patient makes demands on top. In adults this has been found to cause more adverse effects while pain relief is no better. In children a low dose background infusion (4 μg/kg/h) has been found to improve the sleep pattern in the first

24 to 48 hours after surgery without increasing the incidence of adverse effects.

Electronic PCA devices can store data about the way the pump has been used in their memory and this is helpful for assessing the correctness of the programming, when checking for pump malfunctions and to measure morphine consumption.

PCA works best if the patients are selected carefully for their ability to understand and physically operate the pump. Very young children, mentally impaired patients or patients with injuries or burns to their hands are not usually suitable. Children of 5 years and over can usually be taught to operate these devices. Tuition is best carried out in the preoperative period with further encouragement after surgery. Instructions to help mobilization and physiotherapy should be given so that the patient uses the device before trying to move or cough or sit up. PCA should be kept available until the demands drop off.

The amount of morphine which patients require varies by up to a factor of 10. The use of adequate doses of non-steroidal anti-inflammatory drugs (NSAIDs) and/or paracetamol given along with the PCA morphine usually results in a reduced patient need for morphine. This 'morphine-sparing effect' is helpful because side-effects of morphine tend to be dose related, with a lower dose producing fewer side-effects.

Weaning from PCA across to NSAIDs or paracetamol is best judged once the patient is starting to mobilize more actively as morphine requirements may go up at the start of mobilization. Other opioids (e.g. codeine, dihydrocodeine) should not be given to the patient while PCA is running because their effects on breathing will add to those of morphine.

PCA morphine can also be delivered by the subcutaneous route rather than the conventional intravenous route. The subcutaneous route is particularly useful in children and in chronic pain treatment.

The PCA device can be used for nurse-controlled analgesia (NCA). This means that the pump can be programmed to give a continuous infusion of morphine with the nurse giving additional bolus doses when the patient makes a demand. This allows the device to be used in a wider range of patients, for example small children, handicapped patients, patients with hand injuries or burns, the elderly, intensive care patients. This is quite safe provided patients are properly monitored and the nurse knows when *not* to activate the device.

Continuous intravenous infusion of morphine is widely used in intensive care units and can be used safely in general ward areas with appropriate patient monitoring and staffing. The prescription allows the nurse to adjust the infusion rate within limits based upon the monitoring results. This then is a form of nurse-controlled analgesia.

With all opioid infusion techniques, doses must be carefully titrated and individualized for the patient's age, medical condition and surgical procedure. For i.v. opioid infusions or PCA, a separate cannula should be sited and reserved for the opioid infusion. If the same i.v. cannula has to be used for the opioid and other infusions of drugs or fluids, then a valve should be used in the line to stop free-flow by gravity of the opioid into the patient and to prevent reflux of the opioid up the other line. The danger in both these cases is of an inadvertent bolus overdose of opioid. The effect of gravity free-flow (also known as siphonage) is also limited if pumps are mounted horizontally and less than one metre above the patient.

Opioids can also be delivered by infusion or bolus doses into the epidural space. Low doses, added to bupivacaine, result in prolonged pain relief. Higher doses can produce adverse effects noted below. If morphine is given epidurally, some is absorbed into the cerebrospinal fluid. As this fluid circulates slowly over many hours, a small amount of morphine can be carried to the brain and produce late ventilatory depression.

Adverse effects of opioids

All opioids produce dose-related depression of consciousness and breathing. These adverse effects must be regularly assessed as they are potentially life threatening. The level of sedation should be regularly checked and is a sensitive early warning sign of overdosage with morphine. Counting the respiratory rate is often taught as a good sign of opioid-induced ventilatory depression but it is a late sign. Measuring the arterial oxygen saturation by pulse oximetry (SpO_2) is very useful and is particularly sensitive if the patient is breathing room air. As respiratory depression starts to occur, the arterial PCO_2 rises and the SpO_2 starts to fall early. If, however, the patient is breathing added oxygen, the arterial PCO_2 may rise to very high levels before the SpO_2 starts to fall so the SPO_2 is now a late warning sign. In paediatrics, continuous SPO_2 monitoring with the child breathing air is recommended when opioids are used.

Treatment of ventilatory depression consists of stopping the opioid, giving oxygen, supporting the airway and assisting ventilation. In severe cases, the opioid antidote naloxone should be considered (2–100 μg/kg) but administration will usually also reverse analgesia. It is also important to remember that the effects of naloxone do not last very long and in cases of severe opioid overdosage, as might occur if an infusion pump malfunctions, repeated doses of naloxone or a naloxone infusion may be needed. The anaesthetist will decide the need for and dose of naloxone.

Nausea and vomiting are among the most common adverse effects of opioids and can be minimized by using the minimum effective analgesic dose of opioid. If morphine-sparing drugs are used, such as NSAIDs and paracetamol, then the reduced morphine requirement results in less nausea and vomiting. Antiemetic drugs (Table 19.4) can also be used but some produce sedation and other adverse effects such as involuntary movements (particularly in children).

Other adverse effects of opioids including slowing of gut motility, urinary retention and itching. The latter two are more common and severe after epidural opioids.

Other Analgesic Agents

The NSAID group of drugs such as diclofenac, ketorolac and ibuprofen act to inhibit the production of pain-producing substances in the tissues, brain and spinal cord. They are very good for preventing and treating mild and moderate pain and, along with opioids, produce a morphine-sparing effect when treating severe pain.

Paracetamol is a mild analgesic which probably acts on the nitric oxide pain pathway in the brain and spinal cord. It is a very useful drug in paediatrics when given in adequate doses because it is readily available in convenient syrup, suppository and tablet forms.

Weaker opioids such as codeine or dihydrocodeine are also useful for step-across or step-down analgesia. Combinations of paracetamol and codeine are quite effective for moderate pain. Newer opioids such as tramadol and remifentanil are expensive at present but may find a place for specific patients.

Weaning from complex to simple analgesic techniques

Weaning must be individualized depending on monitoring results, mobilization, pain scores, surgical procedure and medical condition. Delay in weaning is most often due to the development of a surgical complication. It is important not to abruptly discontinue a complex technique without giving consideration to step-across analgesia. It is best to have therapeutic levels of alternative drugs established before trying to wean from the complex technique. Beware, however, coprescription of different opioids such as morphine and codeine, as serious ventilatory depression can occur with these combinations. The complex technique should be kept available for a few hours in case it is needed, which helps to reduce patient anxiety about giving up the complex method. The timing of weaning should be judged so as to allow pain-free mobilization.

Table 19.3

ADVERSE EFFECTS OF OPIOIDS

- respiratory depression
- sedation
- nausea
- vomiting
- itching
- urinary retention
- slowing of gut motility
- muscle rigidity/spasms
- allergy
- fall in blood pressure
- tolerance/addiction/withdrawal syndrome

Table 19.4

ANTIEMETICS

- ondansetron
- droperidol
- metoclopramide
- prochlorperazine
- trimeprazine
- hyoscine

20. Preparation for Return to the Ward

E. Holmes

All patients must be assessed prior to their return to the ward. This may be done by the anaesthetist caring for the patient or by a senior nurse within the unit. There should be a unit policy to determine the minimum acceptable criteria for fitness to leave recovery. It is important to take into account the individual needs of the patient and to consider the ward or unit they are being sent to.

Discharge Checklist

- Maintaining own airway
- all protective reflexes returned to normal
- breathing adequately with no evidence of airway obstruction
- SpO_2 >94%, pink, normal respiratory rate
- blood pressure normal
- heart rate and rhythm normal
- perfusion normal (peripheries warm and pink with rapid capillary refill)
- awake and orientated or asleep but responds appropriately to spoken commands
- pain is controlled
- Postoperative Nausea and Vomiting (PONV) is controlled
- local or regional block effective and documented adequately
- fluid balance normalized (i.v. fluids, urinary output, nasogastric and drain losses)
- patient cleaned and linen changed where necessary
- results of investigations available (e.g. X-rays, blood results, urinalysis)
- complications noted
- all documentation filed

When all these details have been reviewed and the decision to transfer the patient has been made, there should be a formal verbal and written handover to the ward staff. The arrangements for transfer and escort to the ward will be decided locally but it is essential that trained staff accompany the patient. The level of electronic monitoring used during the transfer will be individualized and remember that the most important monitor is the trained member of staff. The patient requires constant observation by the escort nurse who must be confident in recognizing signs of ventilatory, circulatory and neurological failure and who must be able to take appropriate action if an emergency arises. Movement of the patient during transfer may cause pain, nausea and vomiting. Bringing the patient's bed to recovery is helpful as the number of moves is then reduced.

There should always be emergency equipment available with the patient which should be checked, in working order and the escort must know how to use the equipment appropriately. Oxygen therapy equipment, self-inflating bag and mask, suction equipment, vomit bowls, tissues, disposal bags, electronic monitors and resuscitation drugs should be carried. The security of infusions, drains and catheters during transfer must be ensured as accidental removal may cause great distress to the patient and may necessitate a further procedure to replace them.

Handover to the Ward Staff

The receiving nurse should assess the patient as in the A–F guide (Chapter 17) and the following information should be passed on at the handover:

- surgical procedure and surgeon
- anaesthetic technique and anaesthetist
- condition and interventions in recovery
- problems
- chart recordings
- drugs given and their effects
- drains, catheters, i.v. sites, fluids
- special requirements
- continuing care needs: fluids, antibiotics, anticoagulant therapy, position, oxygen therapy, pain control.

Key Learning Points

1. The skills and equipment in recovery are similar to those used during the preoperative preparation, induction and maintenance of anaesthesia.

2. Good communication of the details of each individual patient's medical status, surgery and anaesthesia will allow early postoperative problems to be anticipated, identified and treated quickly.

3. Prevention and control of pain should be a high priority in postoperative care.

4. A detailed handover to ward staff using a checklist is essential for patient safety.

Further Reading

'The complete recovery room book'. A Hatfield, M Tronson. Oxford Medical Publications, Oxford, 1992.

'Acute pain management – a practical guide'. PE Macintyre, LB Ready. WB Saunders, London, 1996

'The management of acute pain'. G Park, B Fulton. Oxford Medical Publications Oxford, 1991.

'Patient controlled analgesia'. ML Heath, VJ Thomas. Oxford Medical Publications, Oxford, 1993.

Relevance

ODP Level   Units 4, 7.

SECTION 6
ANAESTHESIA FOR SPECIALTY SURGERY

21. THORACIC, CARDIAC AND VASCULAR SURGERY

D. Paul

This chapter deals, in large part, with anaesthesia for the surgical treatment of smoking related diseases. The patients tend to be middle-aged or older and have mixed pathologies including chronic obstructive airways disease, ischaemic heart disease and peripheral vascular disease. Many vascular patients also have diabetes.

THORACIC SURGERY

The three commonest operations are bronchoscopy, mediastinoscopy and thoractomy.

Bronchoscopy

Bronchoscopy may be performed with a flexible bronchoscope on a sedated patient. There should be i.v. access and nasal or oral oxygen. Monitoring should include ECG, pulse oximeter, BP and verbal contact. The patient normally lies on his side.

Surgical bronchoscopy is usually performed with a rigid bronchoscope and lasts fewer than 10 minutes. The patient lies supine and is anaesthetized and paralysed with short-acting drugs. He is then ventilated by mask until the surgeon intubates the trachea with a ventilating bronchoscopy. This is used with a Sanders' injector which connects directly to the 400 kPa oxygen supply. The injector has a sprung on/off switch which can blast a controllable amount of oxygen through an oblique side-arm of the bronchoscope. This arrangement entrains sufficient air for the oxygen/air mix to inflate the lungs. The bronchoscope is open to air so the gas pressure in the lungs seldom exceeds 30 cmH$_2$O and should never be high enough to cause damage. The patient is kept anaesthetized and paralysed with i.v. boluses. At the end of the procedure the patient is ventilated by mask until breathing and then allowed to waken. If going on to mediastinoscopy, the patient should be intubated with a normal endotracheal tube. Monitoring should include ECG, BP and pulse oximeter.

Mediastinoscopy

Mediastinoscopy and biopsy usually takes about 20 minutes and is performed through a small suprasternal incision. The surgeon stands at the patient's head so the anaesthetic machine and venous access have to be to one side. The monitoring required is standard (ECG, BP and pulse oximeter) but may include a nerve stimulator and CO_2. Problems for the anaesthetist can include profound bradycardia from vagal stimulation and uncontrollable bleeding from large retrosternal vessels.

Thoracotomy

Thoracotomies are most often performed to remove lung tumours by lobectomy or pneumonectomy. Oesophageal and aortic surgery are less common. All are large operations and will last for at least one and a half hours. The problems are the same as for most major surgery but include those of ventilation (see below).

Monitoring will usually include ECG, pulse oximeter, CO_2, nerve stimulator, temperature and an arterial line. Some patients will need a central line. Have available a sheepskin or ripple mattress, heat retaining bonnet, breathing filter, tracheal suction catheters, a fluid warmer and a pressure bag.

The patient is anaesthetized supine in the anaesthetic room. It is often easier to induce and intubate with ECG, BP and pulse oximeter before siting the rest of the monitoring. If this is not then connected until the patient has been positioned in theatre there is less chance of the lines being pulled out. Intravenous line, arterial line and central line should all be sited on the side of the operation. This improves access in theatre and, for a subclavian central line, prevents any complications from a pneumothorax.

In theatre, positioning is important. Have enough people to turn the patient in a controlled way so that lines and the tracheal tube do not become displaced. Once on his side, stop him rolling by placing table brackets across his pelvis anteriorly and sacrum posteriorly. The upper arm should be flexed so that the hand is in front of the face and then raised on an arm rest to allow access to the tracheal tube. The lower arm can be flexed to pass under the chin so that the hand rests by the upper shoulder. Check the brachial plexus is not under tension. Pad all potential pressure areas and include a pillow between knees and ankles. Once the patient is on his side and fully monitored the anaesthetist may wish to insert an epidural catheter or perform intercostal blocks. Anaesthetic problems include blood loss, temperature control and ventilation.

Ventilation

Thoracic anaesthesia is complicated by the fact that it is often necessary to stop ventilating the lung upon which the surgeon is working. It is possible, using a normal tracheal tube, to stop ventilating both lungs for short periods. However, if periods of apnoea longer than 1 or 2 minutes are required it is essential to ventilate each lung separately with a double lumen tube (DLT). There have been many types of DLT but those presently available are either reusable red rubber tubes of Robertshaw design or single use plastic equivalents. They come in a range of sizes and are shaped to intubate the right or left main bronchus. All DLTs have a tracheal and a bronchial lumen, each with an inflatable cuff. A right-sided tube is easily recognised by an aperture in the distal cuff to allow ventilation of the right upper lobe bronchus. Practice varies but most anaesthetists will use a tube for the side opposite the operation.

The patient is anaesthetized and paralysed as normal. The trachea is intubated and the DLT advanced as far as comfortable before inflating the tracheal cuff. The DLT can be positioned clinically by inflating both cuffs and listening to each lung in turn as each lumen is occluded by the assistant using a drain clamp on instructions from the anaesthetist. Clinical positioning is not always reliable so many anaesthetists prefer to check the position with a fibre-optic bronchoscope.

During the operation it is possible to help the surgeon by collapsing the upper lung. This can cause the patient's saturation to decrease to an unacceptable level. The easiest treatment is to insufflate the unventilated lung with 4–6 l/min of oxygen from a standard oxygen cylinder, flow meter, oxygen tubing and suction catheter. The inspired oxygen concentration is usually run at 50–100% depending on the SpO_2 level and blood gas results.

Other Operations

Other relatively short thoracic procedures include oesophagoscopy, insertion of chest drain, talc pleurodhesis and rib resection for empyema. Again, practice varies but these cases are usually intubated and use basic monitoring of ECG, BP and pulse oximeter.

CARDIAC ANAESTHESIA

The two commonest cardiac operations in the UK are coronary artery bypass grafting and heart valve replacement. Both operations use the same anaesthetic set-up. Despite its reputation, much of cardiac surgery and anaesthesia is straightforward. However, this depends very much on the preparation and routine of a well organized theatre. In addition to nurses, orderlies, assistants and medical staff, a cardiac theatre will usually have heart–lung perfusionists and physiological monitoring technicians. Depending on local practice, this latter group may organize all of the peri-operative monitoring.

Basic monitoring for cardiac anaesthesia includes ECG, pulse oximeter, CO_2, arterial line, central line, urine output and core and peripheral temperature. Regular blood gases and activated clotting times are measured in theatre. A pulmonary artery catheter may be used to measure pulmonary artery wedge pressure, cardiac output and oxygen consumption. An extra transducer is sometimes needed to take spot pressures around the heart or to measure left atrial pressure. Rarely, EEG, transoesophageal echo or an aortic balloon pump will be needed. It is probably safe to assume that if something can be measured someone will, at some stage, want to do so.

In addition to the monitoring equipment above, setting up requires a large i.v. cannula and extension set, intubation equipment, a warming or ripple blanket, a reflective bonnet and protecting pressure areas. 'Jelly' pads and rolls are used to protect sacrum and heels. Some patients will need a roll under their shoulders to improve surgical access.

Cardiac patients can decompensate very quickly. It is important to have an emergency drug tray or trolley, defibrillator and pacing box (electrical stimulator for the heart) by the anaesthetic machine in theatre. In addition, there should be i.v. fluids, a pressure bag, syringes, needles, and infusion pumps and their disposables to hand. Sick patients may need extra electrical sockets to cope with the number of pumps. A bucket of ice and water keeps the cardioplegia cold (a solution given into the coronary arteries to protect the heart muscle). With the potential need for so much equipment and monitoring, the top end of the table can become very cluttered and confusing. Many anaesthetists cope by becoming territorial and adhering to set rituals.

Cardiac patients are usually heavily premedicated with benzodiazepines and opiates and often come to theatre breathing oxygen. Some monitoring (usually ECG, arterial line and pulse oximeter) is set up before induction. Once anaesthetized and intubated a central line is inserted and the patient catheterized. In theatre, the sternum is split (with ventilation suspended during the time this is done) and, for bypass grafting, the internal mammary artery and long saphenous vein are dissected out. The patient is heparinized, the aorta and vena cavae cannulated and the patient put on bypass.

Ventilation is then stopped. The heart is isolated from the circulation and then stopped and protected with a cardioplegic solution. Once the grafts or valve are in place, blood is allowed back through the coronary arteries and the heart starts to beat. At this point it may need to be defibrillated or paced. When the heart has settled, the lungs are reventilated and bypass slowly reduced to allow the heart to take over the circulation. This is the stage at which problems are most likely to occur and when drugs and infusions may be needed in a hurry. Once safely off bypass the heparin is reversed with protamine and the patient is closed. The blood left in the heart–lung machine is bagged and reinfused or the red cells can be spun down and washed using a 'cell-saver' device.

At the end of the operation the patient, monitoring, infusions, drains and notes are transferred to a bed and taken to ICU. Many units have a transfer trolley which clips over the bottom of the bed with monitoring, simple ventilator, suction, defibrillator and emergency drugs.

VASCULAR ANAESTHESIA

The commonest vascular procedure is the surgical correction of varicose veins. There are no specific anaesthetic requirements and bleeding is normally minimal. Most patients will have a general anaesthetic although many will receive a regional block with light sedation. The remaining patients that require vascular surgery tend to be older than those with varicose veins and to be less fit. Many have been smokers and suffer varying degrees of peripheral vascular disease, ischaemic heart disease and chronic bronchitis. A proportion have vascular disease as a complication of diabetes. Anaesthetic techniques for vascular surgery range from general anaesthesia alone through combined general and regional to regional alone. In each case, the monitoring and setting up should be similar as some regional anaesthetics may need to be turned into generals if the proposed area of surgery has to be extended. Vascular cases can be long and since many of the patients have poor peripheral circulation it is vital to protect pressure areas and keep the patient warm. Even a femoral embolectomy performed under local and light sedation can cause problems.

The 'intermediate' revascularizations such as femoropopliteal bypasses, tend not to bleed but may be extended to larger procedures. Monitoring is often straightforward (ECG, BP, CO_2 and pulse oximeter) and seldom requires arterial or central lines.

The largest vascular operations are those for repair or replacement of the thoracic or abdominal aorta. Depending on the site and extent of a thoracic lesion (coarctation or aneurysm) the anaesthetic management will combine aspects of a cardiac bypass and a thoracotomy. An abdominal aneurysm can cause equal problems. All aneurysm surgery should have monitoring comparable to that for cardiac bypass: ECG, pulse oximeter, CO_2, arterial line, central line, urine output and core and peripheral temperature. A pulmonary artery catheter may be needed. There is the potential for massive blood loss so large i.v. cannulae, pressure infusors, a blood warmer and a warming blanket are essential. Blood cross-matching forms and tubes should be in theatre along with syringes for measuring blood gases and a means of measuring the activated clotting time. Several infusion pumps and disposables should be available for inotropes, renal dopamine and vasodilators to help control blood pressure and cardiac output. At the end of the surgery the patient should be transferred to a HDU or ITU.

Some patients have sufficiently diseased carotid arteries to require an endarterectomy (coring out the diseased lining of the carotid artery). The anaesthetic problems are lack of access to the head and neck, a very labile blood pressure with manipulation of both the carotid sinus and vagus nerve and the possibility of the patient having a peri-operative stroke. Most anaesthetists would use a standard, ventilated anaesthetic and ask the surgeon to block the carotid sinus with local anaesthetic. Monitoring includes CO_2, an arterial line and, perhaps, an EEG to detect changes in brain activity at the time of carotid clamping.

Amputation

Limbs with end-stage peripheral vascular disease become gangrenous, at which point amputation is the only treatment. Since regional anaesthesia relieves the severe pain of ischaemia and provides good postoperative pain relief many leg amputations are performed under spinal or epidural anaesthesia. Patients must be well enough sedated to be amnesic for the event. Monitoring should include ECG, BP and pulse oximeter.

22. HEAD AND NECK SURGERY

M. McNeil

All forms of surgery involving the patients head and neck result in some special requirements, regardless of which specific surgical specialty is performing. Plastic surgeons, ENT surgeons, maxillofacial surgeons or general surgeons can all produce specific problems for the anaesthetist by virtue of the fact that they are operating in and around the airway.

THE SHARED AIRWAY

Normally the anaesthetist has the luxury of uninterrupted access to the patient's airway and can check on the endotracheal tube and make adjustments as necessary. When surgery is being carried out in this area, it becomes impossible to make any modifications without disturbing the sterile surgical field. It becomes vital to ensure that the tube is in the correct position and that it is reliably secured in that position in a manner that does not encroach on the surgical field, yet will not be disrupted by the surgery or the preparation of the sterile field.

Intraoral work may also require the insertion of a throat pack to prevent blood and debris soiling the patient's pharynx. There should be a system to record that a throat pack has been inserted and, more importantly, that it has been removed before the patient leaves theatre.

The site and nature of the surgery will determine whether an oral or a nasal endotracheal tube is required. Modern preformed tubes are streamlined and allow the bulky connections to catheter mounts and breathing circuit tubing to be mounted away from the operating site. This will not only improve access for the surgeon but will it more difficult for accidental disconnections to occur. In this area of surgery, the anaesthetist must communicate with the surgeon beforehand to ensure that the set-up satisfies both parties. There is little point in struggling with a difficult nasal intubation if an oral intubation would be easier to perform and would still provide acceptable surgical access.

The nature of head and neck surgery determines that a significant number of patients will have difficult airways and be difficult to intubate. These patients should be anaesthetized with extreme caution. Muscle relaxants must never be given until the airway has been secured. Awake fibreoptic intubation is now the technique of choice for tracheal intubation. However, the nature of the surgery may require the performance of a tracheostomy. If so, this could be performed under local anaesthesia with sedation before anaesthesia is induced. A more detailed account of the management of the difficult airway is included in Chapter 3.

23. PLASTIC SURGERY

M. McNeil

Plastic surgery encompasses a wide variety of surgical procedures in patients of all ages. The workload varies from the removal of lumps and bumps under local infiltration to major reconstructive work requiring microvascular flaps.

Much of the surgery can be performed under regional or local anaesthesia, with or without general anaesthesia. Regional anaesthesia is discussed in Ch. 4 and will not be covered in detail in this chapter. Similarly, the problems of young children requiring surgery are detailed in Ch. 30.

BURNS

A significant proportion of plastic surgical workload will be devoted to patients who have suffered burns. The problems that these patients pose can be divided into two groups: the immediate and the long term. The immediate problems associated with burns are related to the massive loss of body fluid that occurs through the burned skin and to the associated problems caused by smoke inhalation. There is a significant mortality for the more seriously burned patients and others may require intensive care before they are fit enough for surgery. In some centres the burns may be treated by early, radical surgery in the hope of preventing long-term scarring. Early surgery results in very large losses of blood and the anaesthetist should be prepared for this situation. A major problem may be venous access, as most of the normal sites for peripheral cannulation may be burned. The anaesthetist may have to site a large bore central line or intraosseous line, or the surgeon may have to perform a 'cut-down' onto a vein.

The skin normally acts as a barrier to infection and once this barrier is burned the body is extremely vulnerable to infection. Great care must be taken to prevent contamination of any cannulae. The burned patient will also respond abnormally to muscle relaxants. They will be resistant to the effects of non-depolarizing muscle relaxants and except very soon after the burn injury, should never be given suxamethonium, as this can produce an acute rise in the level of serum potassium, which can be fatal.

Microvascular Work

The use of the operating microscope has allowed surgeons to greatly extend the scope and scale of their surgical intervention. Much larger areas of tissue can be resected than was the case in the past, and the resultant deficit can be filled with tissue taken from elsewhere on the body and grafted into place. The survival of this grafted tissue depends on the provision of a satisfactory blood supply through the artery and vein that accompany the graft. The major determinant of the adequacy of the flow through these vessels is the surgical technique. The better the anastamosis, the better the flow to the graft. However, the anaesthetic technique can significantly alter the flow through the vessel. There are several factors which will significantly alter the blood flow through the graft. Cardiac output must be maintained to ensure adequate perfusion of all vital organs as well as the graft. The peripheral vascular resistance can be reduced by vasodilating drugs. These drugs will relax smooth muscle in the wall of the blood vessels, allow then to expand and increase the amount of flow through them.

These blood vessels are also sensitive to the effects of temperature and the level of carbon dioxide in the blood. A decrease in temperature or in the level of carbon dioxide in the blood (produced by altering the level of ventilation) will cause the vessels to constrict. Both parameters should be kept within normal limits.

The anaesthetist must therefore pay meticulous attention to the temperature of the patient and the temperature of the theatre; all indices of cardiovascular function must be maintained at normal levels (BP, heart rate, urine output, CVP), the degree of ventilation closely monitored by measuring the end-tidal CO_2, and blood loss accurately measured and replaced.

Regional anaesthesia may have a role to play in these procedures.

Hypotensive Anaesthesia

Hypotensive anaesthesia is often used in the plastic surgical unit. It is a technique which must be used only by anaesthetists and surgeons who are able to take advantage of the benefits it can provide. The anaesthetist allows the patient's blood pressure to fall well below normal limits for the patient by administering powerful vasoactive agents along with the anaesthetic agents.

The proposed benefits for hypotensive anaesthesia are essentially that it will reduce the amount of blood in the surgical field and thus: (a) it will reduce total blood loss and the requirement for transfusion; (b) it will improve the operating conditions for the surgeon; and (c) by reducing the need for diathermy, it will reduce the amount of dead tissue left behind and reduce the risk of infection.

The main danger is that by reducing the blood pressure, the anaesthetist may be reducing the blood supply to vital organs and putting the patients health or even their life at risk. There are several techniques that can be used in combination to improve the results of hypotensive anaesthesia. The posture of the patient can be altered to raise the site of surgery above the heart. This will reduce the pressure of the blood perfusing the site and will also encourage venous drainage of the area. Care must be taken to prevent venous obstruction developing. Regional anaesthesia will produce a sympathetic block and can reduce the pressure in the blood vessels perfusing the operating site. Vasoactive drugs can be given either alone or in combinations. These agents have profound effects on the cardiovascular system and should be used with great caution. Non-invasive blood pressure monitoring will not detect the rapid changes in pressure that can be produced by these agents, so arterial lines are mandatory. If profound levels of hypotension are required, there may also be a case for monitoring the brain. The electrical activity of the brain can be detected and analysed. Changes in the waveform of this activity can warn the anaesthetist that the pressure is becoming too low. The technique of hypotensive anaesthesia should be performed only by anaesthetists who are experts, on patients who will come to no harm from the technique, and for surgeons who will make the most of the benefits provided.

24. MAXILLOFACIAL SURGERY

M. McNeil

Maxillofacial surgery is surgery to the bones and the skull. The indications for the surgery can vary from trauma, to congenital malformations to cosmetic surgery. The trauma patients can often present problems because of the effects of the tissue damage on their airway. Furthermore, there is sometimes an underlying head injury which, of course, must be treated as the number one priority. Many of these injuries are associated with alcohol abuse, road traffic accidents and assault. The anaesthetist must carefully assess the airway with particular attention to any limitation in mouth opening, which can commonly result from fractures to the facial bones. Awake fibreoptic intubation may be the safest technique of intubating these patients.

Patients with congenital malformations requiring maxillofacial surgery will often have problematic airways. Again, awake fibreoptic intubation is the safest option. The airway is often improved as a result of the surgery, but the patients will require close observation in the immediate postoperative period. On occasions, the patients jaws will be wired together to allow the facial bones to heal in the correct position. These patients must be monitored continuously in the recovery period. Antiemetics should be given prophylactically to prevent the patient vomiting, wire cutters should be available to release the fixation and the staff should be familiar with how to use the cutters in an emergency.

25. DENTAL SURGERY

M. McNeil

Dental chair anaesthesia is primarily performed on children who require dental extractions and are unable to tolerate local anaesthesia. The practice of dental chair anaesthesia has been the subject of considerable controversy following some well publicized, tragic fatal accidents. Sadly, these cases have illustrated areas of practice that are quite unacceptable. Certainly, there is no justification for the anaesthetic and surgery being performed by the same individual. Similarly, it is quite unthinkable that a child could be given a general anaesthetic in a location which has inadequate monitoring or resuscitation facilities. These and other issues have been addressed by the Poswillo Report which has clearly recommended that dental general anaesthetics are given by anaesthetists in fully equipped units.

Dental chair anaesthesia is the extreme example of anaesthetist and surgeon sharing the airway. Extraction of teeth can be performed by the dental surgeon operating in the mouth, while the anaesthetist supports the jaw and holds a nasal mask through which the patient breaths oxygen and anaesthetic gases. This arrangement is only satisfactory for straightforward extractions of a few teeth.

More prolonged surgery will require a more secure airway, either in the form of a laryngeal mask or a tracheal tube.

These procedures are generally carried out as day procedures. The staff must confirm that the child has been fasted and is accompanied by a responsible adult who is able to provide consent.

Induction of anaesthesia can be problematic due to the age of the child and the absence of sedative premedication. Intravenous induction of anaesthesia is a more attractive proposition since the advent of the short acting agent propofol and if there is adequate time, EMLA or Ametop cream, will make venepuncture painless. Inhalation induction of anaesthesia may be difficult if the child refuses to cooperate. The parent can remain with the child during this process to provide reassurance. Halothane or sevoflurane can be used for inhalational induction. Halothane will sensitize the heart to produce dysrhythmias in the presence of circulating adrenaline. Isoflurane is less suitable for inhalational induction because of its pungency which can result in coughing, breath-holding and laryngospasm. It is, however, a better agent for maintenance of anaesthesia because it does not cause arrythmias. Sevoflurane provides very rapid, smooth induction with rapid recovery, a lower incidence of cardiac rhythm abnormalities but is much more expensive. Local anaesthetic blocks given by the anaesthetist or surgeon greatly improve the quality of recovery.

At the end of surgery, the child must be turned into the recovery position and oxygen administered. These children will recover very quickly from the short anaesthetic and will soon be ready to go home.

26. EAR, NOSE AND THROAT SURGERY

C. J. Runcie

GENERAL PRINCIPLES

Nose and throat operations are carried out on the upper respiratory tract. The airway is therefore shared between the surgeon and the anaesthetist. The anaesthetist must preserve a clear airway while allowing the surgeon adequate access and must also prevent soiling of the trachea and lungs with blood and debris.

Intubation of the trachea with specialized tracheal tubes is often required. In patients with diseased airways, intubation may be difficult. Following induction of anaesthesia, complete airway obstruction is more likely in these patients and it may be impossible to relieve this by intubation. To avoid this life-threatening sequence of events, some patients with laryngeal disease may require awake intubation or even tracheostomy under local anaesthesia.

ENT surgery is increasingly carried out on a day-case basis. Premedication may be impossible or inadequate. The anaesthetic assistant has an important role to play in reassuring the patient and reducing anxiety before induction.

SPECIFIC OPERATIONS

Tonsillectomy

The standard anaesthetic technique for this operation involves tracheal intubation, usually with a curved preformed tube. These are C-shaped so that the tracheal tube curves away from the roof of the mouth, giving the surgeon access to the tonsils. A throat pack is not used. Extubation is performed with the patient slightly head down in a lateral position *after full protective reflexes have returned*. An alternative to intubation is the flexible laryngeal mask. When well positioned, these will protect the airway from blood coming from above but many anaesthetists regard this technique as controversial especially in children.

The Postoperative Bleeding Tonsil

Surgery is performed only after adequate resuscitation. Blood from the tonsil bed is usually swallowed. The patient thus has a full stomach and a rapid sequence induction with cricoid pressure is necessary. Intubation may be difficult because of blood in the throat or swelling.

Direct Laryngoscopy/Microlaryngoscopy

Patients having these operations have laryngeal pathology and airway maintenance and intubation may be difficult. To allow surgical access, microlaryngoscopy tubes of internal diameter 5–5.5 mm are used. These are flexible and a stilette may be required.

A medical laser may be used during microlaryngoscopy; potential problems include ignition of the tracheal tube and airway fires. Specialized anaesthetic technique may include the LMA, jet ventilation using the Sanders injector and continuous propofol infusions or a nasopharyngeal airway.

Laryngectomy

This is performed for laryngeal carcinoma; difficult intubation is common and so all necessary equipment should be to hand. An armoured tube with a spiral of metallic wire to prevent kinking is preferred. If dissection of the neck is also performed, the surgeon may ask that the BP be lowered with drugs (induced hypotension). Significant bleeding from large blood vessels in the neck may necessitate transfusion of large volumes of blood. Blood warmers, warming blankets and monitoring of direct arterial and central venous pressures may all be necessary.

Nasal Operations

The anaesthetic technique is similar to that for tonsillectomy except that throat packs are used to catch blood and debris. These *must* be removed at the end of the operation and theatre staff should develop a routine to ensure this. The simplest answer is to tie the pack to the tracheal tube before surgery begins. The flexible LMA plus throat pack is also a suitable technique but is not accepted by all anaesthetists as standard practice.

Middle Ear Surgery

Induced hypotension may be necessary and thus monitoring of direct arterial pressure. Nitrous oxide diffuses into the middle ear and can dislodge surgical grafts. O_2/air is therefore more satisfactory than O_2/N_2O as the carrier gas; air supplies (piped/cylinder) should be available.

27. EYE SURGERY

C. J. Runcie

GENERAL PRINCIPLES

Eye surgery can be performed under either local or general anaesthesia. Traditionally, local anaesthesia has been given by the surgeons, but anaesthetists are increasingly involved.

General anaesthesia presents two main areas of concern. Firstly, patients having cataract operations are often elderly and may have numerous chronic illness. Preoperative assessment must be thorough; anaesthesia must be given meticulously an patiently. Cataract operations are increasingly done as day-case procedures and this may make preoperative assessment difficult. Rapid recovery is important but difficult to achieve in elderly patients with reduced capacity to metabolize drugs.

Control of Intraocular Pressure

The anaesthetist's other main concern is to provide good operating conditions. If the operating microscope is in use, complete immobility of the eye is essential. Intraocular pressure (IOP) must also be controlled and preferably reduced. Once the eye is open, any increase in IOP will push the contents of the eye out through the wound with disastrous results.

Several factors regulate IOP; anaesthetists can most easily influence the choroidal vascular volume (the volume of blood in the arteries and veins of the eye). Arterial hypoxia and hypercapnia increase choroidal vascular volume and thus IOP. Coughing and vomiting increase venous pressure and cause marked increases in IOP. Most anaesthetic drugs reduce IOP, including the induction and inhalational agents and the opiates. Suxamethonium produces a transient rise in IOP.

SPECIFIC OPERATIONS

Intraocular surgery

Standard techniques for intraocular surgery involve tracheal intubation and mechanical ventilation with the inhalational agents to produce mild hypocapnia and ensure good oxygenation. An alternative is mechanical ventilation via the flexible LMA, but only if good position and low airway pressures can be achieved. Continuous infusion of propofol is feasible with the aim of improving recovery. A peripheral nerve stimulator is essential so that neuromuscular function does not recover unexpectedly as coughing and loss of eye contents may result.

The Penetrating Eye Injury

This is problematic as the patient may have eaten just before the injury and thus have a full stomach. Suxamethonium is part of the rapid sequence induction employed in such circumstances but causes a transient rise in IOP which may lead to loss of ocular contents. Some anaesthetists therefore modify the rapid sequence induction in this situation. For most, the good intubating conditions obtained with suxamethonium outweigh the risks.

Extraocular Surgery

The only common operation is squint surgery, which is more painful post-operatively than intraocular surgery. Spontaneous respiration via the LMA is a suitable technique.

The OculoCardiac Reflex

Traction on the eye muscles or pressure on the eyeball can stimulate the vagus and lead to bradycardia or asystole. Treatment is with i.v. atropine or glycopurronium. These should always be readily available for eye surgery.

28. NEUROSURGERY

D. Walker

PROCEDURES

Cranial:
- craniotomies
- posterior fossa operations
- burr holes
- shunts
- others, e.g. cranioplasty.

Spinal:
- cervical
- thoracic/lumbar.

Radiology/imaging and other diagnostic procedures.
Procedures involve both adult and paediatric patients.

GENERAL

The central nervous system is metabolically very active and is readily damaged by episodes of ischaemia which would not cause permanent injury to other organs. Already injured neural tissue is even more susceptible to further damage by otherwise minor episodes of hypoxaemia or reduced perfusion. The aim of neuroanaesthesia is therefore firstly to provide anaesthesia (analgesia and lack of awareness) to enable the surgical procedure to be performed, secondly to optimize operating conditions for the surgeon and thirdly to minimize the potential of adverse effects (particularly ischaemia) in the perioperative period.

CRANIOTOMY

A craniotomy is the removal of a piece of skull to allow surgical access to the intracranial contents.

Nature of procedure

Craniotomies are performed for a number of reasons:

1. clipping of an intracerebral arterial aneurysm
2. removal of all or part of an intracranial tumour
3. removal of an intracranial haematoma and/or damaged brain
4. other procedures, for example resection of an epileptic focus or decompression of a cranial nerve.

Specific Problems

1. Aneurysms: minimizing risk of rupture of aneurysm by preventing rises in blood pressure and maintaining normocapnia.
2. Tumours: maintaining adequate arterial perfusion by minimizing rises in intracranial pressure and keeping an adequate arterial blood pressure.
3. Haematoma: maintaining adequate cerebral perfusion as above, minimizing brain swelling and avoiding hypotension.
4. Some procedures may involve preoperative identification of specific brain structures with electrophysiological equipment.

Anaesthetics – Preparation and Techniques

Anaesthetic machine and ventilator in anaesthetic room and theatre suite checked and operational.

Blood cross-matched and available and checked (2–6 units or more as appropriate).

Trolleys and appropriate equipment prepared for:

- intravenous access, fluid administration and blood warming. (Cannulae, fluids, (giving sets, blood warmer, extension tubing)
- appropriate sized endotracheal tubes, catheter mount and HME/bacterial filter, anaesthetic hoses of adequate length in theatre. Endotracheal tubes are usually secured with adhesive tape, rather than tied in, since tape around the neck may obstruct jugular venous drainage and will obstruct surgical access for cervical procedures
- arterial and central venous pressure monitoring, (cannulae and CVP catheters, fluid, giving set, pressure bag, transducer and pressure tubing)
- urinary catheterization (urinary catheter, measuring/collecting bag)
- spinal drain (epidural set, tubing and collecting bottle).

Anaesthetic Preparation

- Drugs: the anaesthetist will have prepared and checked the drugs required including induction agent, muscle relaxant, analgesia, maintenance agents, vasoactive and emergency drugs, antibiotics.
- Pre-induction: hand over of patient from reception, pre-op checking and transfer to anaesthetic room.
- Pre-induction monitoring – usually at least ECG, NIBP, pulse oximetry and sometimes intra-arterial pressure monitoring, especially in patients with aneurysms.
- Preoxygenation and induction of anaesthesia, intubation, securing of ET tube using adhesive tape, protection of eyes.
- Following intubation, the patient will usually be ventilated mechanically during the insertion of i.v., arterial cannula, spinal drain, urinary catheter and temperature probe as appropriate. Full anaesthetic monitoring continuous during these procedures
- The hair is usually shaved and the skin prepared with antiseptic solutions by the surgeon.

Transfer and Maintenance

The patient, once fully prepared, is moved to the operating theatre, ventilation being continued manually during transfer, and positioned on the operating table. The patient may be supine, lateral, prone or sitting to facilitate surgical access. In all cases, pressure points must be well protected and excessive strain on joints and traction on nerves avoided by keeping joints in as near to a natural position as possible. Facial positioning, which may involve immobilizing the head of a 3-pin head rest, will be done by the surgeon.

Full monitoring is recommended in theatre.

Preoperative

Neurosurgical procedures may be prolonged: vaporizers may need refilling and soda lime canisters changing during the course of the procedure rather than between cases. Blood loss may be minimal, or sudden and substantial. Changes in the patient's temperature may require attention to the theatre temperature.

At the End of the Procedure

Most neurosurgical patients will be woken and extubated at the end of the procedure. Exceptions may include patients with severe head trauma who may be electively ventilated as part of the management of raised intracranial pressure. However, the majority of patients will have residual neuromuscular block reversed at the end of the operation and be extubated as normal once they started breathing and regained protective airway reflexes.

Postoperative

Following a craniotomy, patients should be taken to a recovery ward, high dependency unit, or intensive care unit for close monitoring of their neurological status in the postoperative period, in order that any deterioration can be rapidly detected and managed as appropriate.

29. Assistance in Maternity Hospitals

M. McNeil

Introduction

Anaesthesia for the pregnant woman poses a number of unique problems for the anaesthetist. Firstly, the presence of the fetus means that any intervention to the mother may have an effect on the fetus. Secondly, pregnancy is associated with profound changes in the mother's cardiovascular and respiratory systems, which will alter her response to anaesthetic agents. Thirdly, childbirth is a highly emotional experience for the mother and her partner. A great deal of sensitivity and understanding will be required from those attending a woman in labour. These factors may also be compounded by religious or cultural factors which, although unfamiliar to the staff, must be respected. Finally, the obstetric unit may be in a site that is isolated from other units and assistance may be provided by staff who are not dedicated anaesthetic assistants.

The problems of anaesthesia for pregnant woman are continually highlighted in the Report of the Confidential Enquiry into Maternal Deaths. The latest report, covering the years 1985–1987, shows that there were 8 deaths directly related to anaesthesia in this period. Quite clearly the objective of Obstetric Anaesthetists is to reduce this figure to zero. The provision of skilled assistance for the anaesthetist should form a major part of any scheme to reduce maternal mortality attributable to anaesthesia.

Effect of Anaesthetic on the Fetus

Any drug given to a pregnant woman will have some effect on her unborn child. In the early part of the pregnancy the fetus is developing rapidly. Many drugs given at this stage, before the development of the organs is complete, can produce severe malformations (teratogenesis), the most infamous example of this being the thalidomide tragedy. For this reason, non-urgent surgery should be avoided during the first three months of pregnancy.

Towards the end of the pregnancy, the teratogenic effects of drugs are no longer an issue. However, any drug, given to the mother, including anaesthetic agents, can cross the placenta and adversely affect the baby.

Physiological Changes Associated with Pregnancy

As pregnancy develops, the demands of the fetus for nourishment and oxygen will have to be met by the mother. Her cardiovascular and respiratory system have to increase their workload to cope with these demands. The cardiac output rises from very early on in the pregnancy, the heart rate rises and the blood pressure tends to fall slightly. The rate of breathing is increased and the degree of reserve capacity in the lungs is markedly reduced.

The gastrointestinal system will also be affected. The production of acid by the stomach is increased, and the efficiency of the lower oesophageal sphincter is reduced, thus increasing the likelihood of gastric acid being regurgitated.

Finally, the production of haemoglobin by the mother is increased during pregnancy. However the production of plasma proteins is increased by an even greater degree and, as a result, the actual concentration of haemoglobin in the blood will fall.

Anaesthesia for Caesarean Section

Practical Assistance

Before discussing the different techniques available for anaesthesia there are some practical principles which should be established.

Firstly, the anaesthetic assistant should have no other duties to perform and should always be instantly available.

Secondly, a pregnant woman with an established regional block will have no control over the lower half of her body. She will require to be lifted onto the theatre table. This can be a considerable undertaking and will require the assistance of every available able bodied person in theatre. Drips, urinary catheters and epidural catheters must be safeguarded during the transfer process. On the table, she must be positioned with a lateral tilt to prevent hypotension due to the womb pressing on the inferior vena cava which reduces cardiac output and she must *never* be left unattended.

The standards of intraoperative monitoring for a Caesarean section (whether under regional or general anaesthesia) should be no less rigorous than for a major, elective surgical procedure. ECG electrodes, blood pressure cuff and pulse oximeter should be positioned as soon as the patient is in theatre.

The anaesthetic assistant must be familiar with the layout of the theatre, the location of emergency equipment (blood warmer, CVP lines, intubation aids, etc), and the controls of the operating table and be able to safely move the mother into the lithotomy position.

Regional Anaesthesia

Regional anaesthesia has many advantages over general anaesthesia. The mother can remain awake, can see her child being born and can immediately start the bonding process. Her partner can also participate in the process. The risks of general anaesthesia are avoided, as is the problem of awareness.

Epidural or Spinal Anaesthesia

Epidural or spinal anaesthesia provide the most flexible way for dealing with Caesarean sections. An epidural may already be in position for pain relief in labour, can easily be topped up for the section, and then used to provide postoperative analgesia.

The degree of epidural block required for Caesarean section is greater than for pain relief in labour. Larger doses of local anaesthetic are required than for labour pain control and these must be given carefully, in divided doses, closely observing the patient for signs of toxicity (metallic taste in mouth, ringing in ears, drowsiness, etc).

Spinal anaesthesia produces a much quicker, more profound block and is useful in emergencies. The combination of spinal and epidurals (quick onset; postoperative pain control) is becoming more popular.

The commonest side-effect is hypotension. This is caused by blocking the sympathetic nerve fibres resulting in a direct lowering of blood pressure and also encouraging pooling of blood in the dilated veins of the legs. These effects can be minimized by: avoiding the supine position which causes the enlarged uterus to compress the aorta and inferior vena cava (aortocaval occlusion) thus preventing blood returning to the heart; secondly 'preloading' the circulation with a litre of balanced salt solution will counteract the hypotension; finally intravenous ephedrine (a sympathetic stimulant) can restore the blood pressure.

PAIN RELIEF IN LABOUR

A small percentage (no more than 2%) of women experience little or no pain during labour. For the rest, the degree of pain experienced will vary enormously. There are a wide variety of pain relief techniques available to the mother and she should be encouraged to use techniques with which she is most comfortable.

Antenatal classes allow the mother to get an introduction to the labour ward and to the methods of analgesia available. Relaxation classes can allow the mother and her partner to practice techniques that help her cope with the pain of her contractions without medication. For a fortunate few, this may be all that is required.

For others further analgesia is necessary, and the first step is commonly the use of Entonox. This is a mixture of 50% nitrous oxide in oxygen which is inhaled during the contraction. The characteristics of nitrous oxide are such that its analgesic action has a rapid onset and offset. Entonox can be used in conjunction with other agents such as opiate analgesics. Opiates have long been used in obstetric practice and can be given intramuscularly to provide additional pain relief. Opiates will cross the placenta and will depress the newborn baby's breathing efforts. For this reason, the injection should not be given if the delivery of the baby is expected within 4 hours. Both Entonox and opiates will make the mother drowsy and approximate 50% of mothers consider that the analgesia provided by these agents is unsatisfactory.

Epidural anaesthesia is the most powerful method of pain relief in labour. It is particularly recommended for those women who are at a higher than normal risk of an instrumental delivery. The actual technique of epidural cannulation has been described elsewhere, but one should remember that the mother may be distressed and be unable to keep still during the procedure. Furthermore 'the bump' may prevent the patient from adopting the ideal position for epidural cannulation. Despite this, it is crucial that the mother is assisted into the correct position, with the lower back curled away from the anaesthetist. If this position is not achieved, the insertion of the epidural catheter will be more difficult for the anaesthetist and the mother. Epidural analgesia can provide almost complete relief of pain during labour without making the mother or the baby drowsy. The effect of the block can be extended to allow more invasive procedures to be performed with minimal discomfort.

The disadvantages of epidural analgesia are:

1. An anaesthetist must site the epidural and be available to deal with any complications arising.
2. The epidural can produce weakness of the legs and a sensation of helplessness in the mother. She may require assistance in moving about the bed and should be prevented from adopting postures that will inadvertently strain muscles or ligaments.

3. If the epidural is continued throughout the second stage of labour, there may be an increased chance of a forceps delivery.
4. Large doses of local anaesthetic are required to achieve a block that is adequate for a Caesarean section. Toxic reactions to the local anaesthetic are possible.
5. The epidural catheter may migrate beyond the dura mater and produce an unexpected spinal block.
6. There is a small chance of producing a dural puncture with the risk of subsequent headache.

Spinal anaesthesia will provide effects that are broadly similar to the effects of an epidural anaesthetic. The differences are that: (a) as the drug is administered directly into the CSF, a much smaller dose is required and therefore there is almost no possibility of toxic reaction to the local anaesthetic; and (b) the onset of the block is much more rapid. Consequently, the development of side-effects related to the block are much more rapid in onset and can be more difficult to treat

Spinal anaesthesia is a one-shot technique and the dose cannot be modified at a later time.

As a consequence of a spinal block, a small hole is made in the dura mater through which CSF can leak. This leakage can lower the pressure of the CSF supporting the brain and produce a headache which typically is aggravated by standing. This complication occurs much more commonly in the obstetric population than in general surgical patients, although the incidence has been considerably reduced by the use of pencil point spinal needles. This headache can be effectively relieved by the use of an epidural blood patch, in which 20–20 ml of the patient's own blood is injected into the epidural space, allowing the clot to plug the hole in the dura.

GENERAL ANAESTHESIA

General anaesthesia for the pregnant woman at term can be one of the greatest challenges for the anaesthetist. The pregnant woman at term is at much greater risk of developing hypoxia than her non-pregnant sister due to physiological changes that increase her oxygen consumption yet reduce her oxygen reserves. The risk of regurgitation of gastric contents is also much higher. At the same time, the anaesthetist must carefully control the dosage of anaesthetic agents given to the mother as these affect the newborn baby and, in the case of volatile anaesthetic agents, cause the uterine muscle to relax,

thus increasing the risk of blood loss. Having read the above, it is hardly sur-
prising that the preferred technique for Caesarean section is now regional
anaesthesia.

The vast majority of maternal deaths attributable to anaesthesia are due to
either failure to intubate the trachea or aspiration of gastric contents. The
anaesthetic technique must:

- minimize the risk of hypoxaemia developing
- secure the airway rapidly
- minimize the risk of gastric contents being aspirated
- ensure adequate maternal anaesthesia while preventing neonatal depression
- maintain uterine muscle tone.

Any patient undergoing operative delivery should be given treatment to
reduce the acidity of her gastric contents. This can either be done by H_2
receptor antagonist or by sodium citrate given by mouth shortly before the
start of surgery.

Prophylaxis should be given even if a regional technique is planned, as the
need to give a general anaesthetic may arise without warning.

The patient must be given 100% oxygen to breathe before a rapid sequence
induction is performed. Anaesthesia is induced with thiopentone followed by
suxamethonium. Once the patient is asleep, cricoid pressure is applied. The
cricoid cartilage sits below the thyroid cartilage and is the only cartilage
around the larynx which forms a complete ring. Backward pressure on this
cartilage will therefore be transmitted backwards and compress the oesophagus against the vertebral bodies behind it. This acts as a pinch valve and will
prevent active vomiting and should not be used in that situation. All other
laryngeal cartilage's have soft ligaments at their backs which will not compress the oesophagus. The pressure should be applied in such a way that it
does not interfere with the handle of the laryngoscope. The pressure should
be applied as the woman starts to lose consciousness. If applied too early, it
can provoke coughing and retching. It should be withdrawn only when
the trachea has been intubated, the cuff inflated and an air-tight seal in the
trachea demonstrated.

More simply, the pressure should be maintained until the anaesthetist
instructs otherwise.

If the anaesthetist encounters difficulty in intubating the trachea he must
have a present plan to deal rapidly and efficiently with the situation. This
'Failed Intubation Drill' or one of its modifications should be known by

anyone who is asked to give a general anaesthetic or assist at a general anaesthetic in a maternity hospital.

Pregnancy-induced Hypertension (pre-eclampsia)

This syndrome causes high blood pressure which may be complicated by brain swelling, convulsions, bleeding, heart failure, and kidney failure. Treatment is by correcting all these as far as possible using vasodilators, anticonvulsants, coagulation factors and intotropic and fluid support. Intensive care management and monitoring principles are very appropriate in severe cases.

Bleeding

Obstetric haemorrhage can be very rapid and severe and requires rapid transfusion of fluids, blood, and blood products via large bore cannulae and rapid warming devices. Sometimes uncrossmatched, O negative blood may have to be given as a life saving measure.

Amniotic Fluid Embolus

The entry of amniotic fluid into the mother's circulation can be devastating leading to cardiac arrest and death. In those who survive, bleeding is a major problem; respiratory failure occurs due to occlusion of the lung circulation and pulmonary oedema and heart failure may occur. Treatment is according to principles of resuscitation and intensive care.

Anaesthetic Assistance in the Maternity Hospital

The Obstetric Anaesthetists Association has recently surveyed the level of assistance provided in maternity hospitals. Of 180 hospitals surveyed, the vast majority used the services of ODAs/ODPs. Only in 40 units was assistance provided by midwives. Quite clearly, the standard of assistance should not vary, whoever provides the service.

The Obstetric Anaesthetists Association has formulated guidelines for the standards of training and competency that should be expected of those who assist the anaesthetist in maternity units. Hopefully, these guidelines will become accepted nationally and help to maintain a standard of excellence which will make a contribution to the continuing fall in maternal deaths associated with anaesthesia.

Further Reading

Moir and Thorburn: Obstetric Anaesthesia and Analgesia. 3rd Edition. Bailliere Tindall. 1986.
Report on the Confidential enquiries into maternal deaths in the United Kingdom 1985–1987.

Mason RA: Anaesthesia Databook. 2nd edition. Churchill Livingstone 1994

30. Paediatric Surgery

N. S. Morton

Children are not small adults. The range of diseases they suffer from is different from adults and the child's physical and psychological responses to these diseases are different. Congenital abnormalities or their complications are often the reason for the child coming into hospital for surgery or for emergency care. The child's smaller size affects the equipment used for anaesthesia and the relatively large surface area of the small child means that heat loss and fluid losses are more of a problem. There are several differences in anatomy, physiology, psychology and pharmacology which have to be considered. All these variations are especially marked in the newborn and especially the premature baby.

Differences in Anatomy

Airway

The child has a relatively large head and a short neck which tends to cause the neck to flex on the trunk when the child is lying flat on his back. The face and lower jaw are small and the tongue is relatively large, which makes viewing the larynx more difficult. Also, the airway tends to become obstructed more easily (Fig 30.1). The floor of the mouth is soft and compressible which means care must be taken when holding the jaw to maintain the airway. Only the bony parts of the lower jaw should be held. Babies less than 6 months of age breathe through their noses and any cause of nasal obstruction is serious. This includes nasogastric tubes, temperature probes or secretions. Some babies are born with nasal obstruction (choanal atresia) and if this involves both sides, then urgent or emergency surgery may be needed. As they breathe out, babies naturally generate positive pressure in the lower airways (auto CPAP) by the vocal cords moving towards the midline during expiration. In respiratory diseases this is exaggerated and the baby is heard to make a 'grunting' sound.

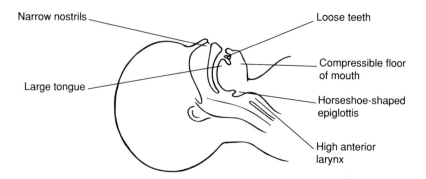

Fig. 30.1 Summary of significant airway anatomy

Lungs

The lungs and airways develop very early in fetal life from 26 to 52 days of gestation and thereafter three main stages are worth noting. From 7 to 16 weeks, airways and lung vessels form, with support cartilage seen from about 10 weeks. Between 16 and 24 weeks, airways continue to grow and a viable gas exchanging surface develops within the lungs. The natural detergent, surfactant, is produced which has the effect of both preventing lung collapse *and* lung over-infiltration. After 24 weeks, there is a huge increase in the gas exchanging surface area to reach the newborn value of 1.8 m². This growth continues after birth for the first 8 years of life until the adult value of about 100 m² is reached.

In utero, the lungs and airways are fluid filled and at birth, the baby takes its first gasps which open up the small airways and gas exchanging sacs (alveoli). The lungs still contain a lot of fluid, but this is gradually absorbed. The newborn baby has to work hard to breathe and any change from normal is not well tolerated.

The oxygen-carrying pigment in the newborn baby's red blood cells (haemoglobin, Hb) is different from that in adults. The baby's haemoglobin, HbF, comprises 70% of the total Hb and cannot release so much oxygen to the tissue cells. This means the baby has less reserves of oxygen supply to the tissues if there are problems with breathing, the child's airway or circulation and so very low oxygen levels in the tissues can occur much more quickly than in adults.

Heart and Circulation

In the fetus before birth, the lungs are collapsed and filled with fluid so the blood flow to the lungs is very low, with nutrient gas exchange occurring by the placenta (between mother and baby).

With the first breath, the lungs expand and blood flow to the lungs increases very quickly. The oxygen level in the arterial blood rises and this causes further relaxation of the lung blood vessels. Blood flow from the lungs via the pulmonary veins also increases and this will cause oxygenated blood to return to the left atrium. The pressure in the left atrium rises and the atrial septum is pushed over like a flap to close off the normal atrial septal hole (foramen ovale) which is present in the fetus.

Another effect of increased oxygen in the arterial blood is to cause narrowing and eventual closure of a vessel known as the arterial duct. This vessel runs between the pulmonary artery and the aorta. It carries the blood which bypasses the unused lungs in the fetus. Once the baby is breathing, however, this vessel is no longer needed as it is important that the lungs now receive their full quota of blood flow. If this vessel does not close off, blood from the higher pressure aorta can flood the lung circulation. This patent arterial duct can be closed by drug treatment (indomethacin), by placing an occluding device using a special catheter or by an open operation to tie off or clip the vessel.

The heart of the newborn baby has relatively few muscle fibres and this means it has less reserves of function to cope with added circulatory stresses. Cardiac output is very dependent on the heart rate and there is a limit to how much the heart rate can increase and how long this increase can be sustained.

Spinal Cord and Epidural Space

In the newborn baby, the spinal cord and dural sac end at a much lower level than in the older child or adult (Fig. 30.2). Thus care must be taken when performing caudal epidural blocks not to puncture the dura and when performing spinal blocks to use the L5/S1 space.

DIFFERENCES IN PHYSIOLOGY

The effects of the differences in anatomy are reflected in differences in function between children and adults. There are lesser reserves of lung function, cardiac and circulatory function and oxygen-carrying capacity and thus any stresses will produce effects more rapidly. The child's metabolic rate is higher than adults and thus oxygen is used up more quickly by cells. The stressed baby reacts by increasing its rate of breathing and increasing the heart rate but eventually cannot sustain these changes and becomes

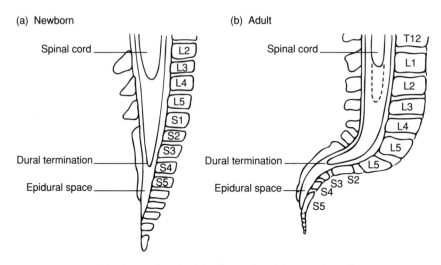

Fig. 30.2 *The spinal cord and dural sac end much lower in the newborn*

exhausted. Breathing rate may then fall and indeed stop. This is an emergency situation as oxygen is used rapidly by the tissues and oxygen supply to the brain and heart fails. The heart rate slows (bradycardia) in response to this fall in oxygen supply.

The large surface area of children in relation to their weight means that heat loss is greater and care must be taken to minimize this as cold puts a considerable additional stress on the cardiovascular and respiratory systems. Covering the baby, warming inspired gases and intravenous fluids, and the use of radiant heaters all help to minimize heat loss.

The liver and kidneys are relatively immature up to the age of three months and 12 months, respectively, and this has important implications for drug dosages (see below) and drug toxicity. The kidneys cannot handle sodium or sugar loads well and care must be taken not to give too high amounts of these compounds in intravenous infusions.

DIFFERENCES IN PHARMACOLOGY

As the liver is relatively immature, it does not produce so many proteins and those drugs which are normally highly bound to proteins will be circulating in their free unbound form. This means that they exert more clinical *and* toxic effects (e.g. bupivacaine). The enzyme systems which break down drugs are immature until about 3 months of age and this results in a prolonged effect from a given dose. This is made worse by the immaturity of the kidneys which clear many drugs from the body after they have been metabolized by the liver. The immaturity of the brain and blood–brain barrier means that small babies are very sensitive to the effects of sedative drugs. A good example to illustrate the differences in drug handling is to consider morphine. The neonatal brain is sensitive to the sedative and respiratory depressant effects of morphine and a given dose will last a long time, with smaller amounts being metabolized by the liver and excreted by the kidney. Thus, the effects of the drug on the child and the child on the drug are quite different from adults.

PAEDIATRIC ASPECTS OF PREOPERATIVE ASSESSMENT AND PREPARATION

Most children undergoing surgery are well, have a single problem (often one they are born with) which requires a relatively minor surgical procedure to correct. Many such children can have their surgery on a day-case basis and it is the selection of cases who are not suitable for this type of care that becomes important.

Other children have more complex congenital abnormalities or multiple abnormalities which need more complex or more invasive anaesthesia, surgery, monitoring and postoperative care.

The age, maturity, surgical procedure and medical condition all have an influence on the anaesthetic technique used.

Nearly all children benefit from parents being present with them while they are conscious and parental presence during induction of anaesthesia is usually to be encouraged. Occasionally, a very anxious parent may be advised not to attend the induction as they will transmit anxiety to their child. Where problems are anticipated during induction of anaesthesia, it may be advisable for the parent not to attend. Avoidance of separation from parents is particularly important for pre-school children and some units also allow parents to be present during the recovery phase.

Premedication with heavy sedation is not required for the majority of children if they are being managed in a child-friendly environment with parents closely involved. However, some children will benefit from sedative premedication, especially those showing signs of anxiety or who are inconsolable. Occasionally, a child will not cooperate with any attempts at consolation and refuses premedication also. This is a difficult situation under the current legislation and the medical staff have to make a judgement about how urgent the surgery is and whether it needs to proceed. Discussion with the parents is helpful also in determining whether an appropriate amount of restraint of the child is acceptable, for example to give an intramuscular injection, to establish venous access or to undertake an inhalational induction of anaesthesia. Intramuscular ketamine can be useful in this difficult situation.

If the child will take a drink then a small volume with midazolam 0.5 mg/kg or ketamine 5 mg/kg is effective in 15–30 minutes.

Preparation of the child for the intravenous induction of anaesthesia will usually include use of a topical local anaesthetic cream applied to the skin, about 1–1.5 hours in advance. EMLA cream, which is a 50:50 mixture of lignocaine and prilocaine, should be used routinely in children except in those under 1 year of age, those with eczema and those with known allergy to local anaesthetics. Infants and eczematous children are at risk of absorbing the local anaesthetics into the blood with a possibility of toxic effects. In practice, many units use EMLA in infants under 1 year of age but it must be prescribed and must only be applied for 1 hour. A new local anaesthetic cream (amethocaine) is due for release soon and has the advantage of a quicker onset of effect (30–40 minutes).

A very important part of the preanaesthetic visit, assessment and preparation of the child is the discussion with the parents, and the child where appropriate, about pain management.

This should cover the techniques planned for use in theatre and postoperatively and should include discussion of the risks, benefits and logic of the methods to be used. Parents often ask for clarification of epidurals, caudals, PCA and the use of morphine. They may have experience of these techniques themselves and may be for or against a particular method.

It is important to discuss the concept of co-analgesia and to mention the role of suppository formulations of analgesia in children. Parents may worry about the suppository route and a clear explanation of the benefits will be helpful. If parents (or children) do not wish a particular technique to be used then this should be respected.

Fasting Guidelines

Prolonged fasting before anaesthesia is unnecessary and can be harmful, especially in small children. Dehydration and hypoglycaemia can occur in infants fasted for long periods and this effect is more evident the younger the child is. The aim is to have a child with an empty stomach but who is not fluid depleted. Any stomach contents should not be too acidic and there should be no solid particles of food. Milk becomes in effect a solid when it enters the stomach, so bottled milk, milk formula baby feeds or milky drinks should be classified as solids for the purposes of fasting rules. Breast milk, however, is cleared relatively quickly from the baby's stomach and a shorter fasting interval is allowed for breast-fed babies. Clear fluids are emptied from the stomach very quickly and so a much shorter period is allowable. Water, fizzy drinks, juices, tea and coffee made with water all classes as 'clear fluids'. Modern fasting guidelines for elective paediatric cases therefore are:

- 6 hours for solids, mil or milky drinks
- 4 hours for breast milk
- 3 hours for clear fluids.

INDUCTION OF ANAESTHESIA IN CHILDREN

The routine use of topical local anaesthetic creams (EMLA or Ametop) in Europe has resulted in more intravenous inductions of anaesthesia in the last few years. The introduction of propofol and the laryngeal mask airway into paediatric practice has also resulted in more i.v. inductions because this technique is so useful for the majority of paediatric operations. Propofol does produce injection pain but this can be reduced by adding lignocaine, 0.2 mg/kg. Intravenous induction can thus be painless and atraumatic for the child if they are told what is to happen, are reassured and a parent is present. An example of how this can work well is to have the child walk along hand in hand with mum into the anaesthetic room where mum sits on a stool or chair with her child on her lap. The anaesthetic room should be made as child-friendly as possible with lots of pictures and cartoons and the assistant can help greatly by striking up a rapport and conversation with the child and parent. EMLA is removed and the child gives their mum a cuddle with one hand round behind mum's neck or back. The anaesthetist can then cannulate this hand out of direct sight and the assistant applies fixing tape or a dressing.

If inhalational induction is used it is important that this is made as atraumatic as possible and a similar approach is taken as with i.v. induction. The anaesthetist disguises the anaesthetic circuit by running it behind the arm and using the cupped hand as the mask. The hand is tucked under the child's chin while the child sits on his parent's lap. The volatile agents halothane or sevoflurane are the best, along with nitrous oxide 67% in oxygen if this is deemed safe. Some older children like the idea of a facemask as a pilot's mask or spaceman's mask and the clear shell masks are much more child-friendly. The parent is warned that the child may go through a short period of excitement or restlessness and it is best to allow relatively free movement as stimulation caused by trying to prevent movement of arms and legs can make the restlessness worse. Once the child is settled they are lifted onto the anaesthetic trolley and the parent is escorted out of the induction room by a member of staff other than the anaesthetic assistant. The assistant applies monitors and helps with venous cannulation.

MAINTENANCE OF ANAESTHESIA IN CHILDREN

The majority of children can be safely managed by a laryngeal mask, spontaneous respiration, local block technique. Otherwise the principles and practice of maintenance of anaesthesia and monitoring are very similar to adult practice. The main differences are in the size of equipment and the doses of drugs used. A local or regional block or wound infiltration with local anaesthetic should be part of the anaesthetic technique for all children unless there is a specific contraindication. Loading doses of opioids, NSAIDs and paracetamol should be given prior to the surgical stimulus where indicated and opioid infusions for postoperative analgesia should be started during anaesthesia.

PAEDIATRIC RESUSCITATION (SEE P. 150)

There are several courses teaching paediatric resuscitation throughout the United Kingdom (e.g. Paediatric Advanced Life Support – PALS). These are well advertised in professional journals.

Further Reading

'Paediatric Day Case Surgery'. NS Morton, PAM Raine. Oxford Medical Publications, Oxford, 1994.
'Handbook of neonatal anaesthesia'. DG Hughes, SJ Mather, AR Wolf. WB Saunders, London, 1996.
'Wylie and Churchill-Davidson's A Practice of Anaesthesia', 6th edition. Edited by TEJ Healy and PJ Cohen. Edward Arnold, London, 1996.
'Case presentations in paediatric anaesthesia and intensive care'. NS Morton, E Doyle. Butterworth Heinemann, Oxford, 1994.

Relevance

ODP Level 3   Units 3, 4, 5, 6, 7, 8.

31. MINIMALLY INVASIVE SURGERY

N. S. Morton

Recently, interest in surgical techniques via telescopic instruments using fibreoptic technology has developed, although some basic techniques and principles have been in use in gynaecology for many years. Laparoscopy is where a fibreoptic light source and imaging system is pushed through a small incision in the abdomen into the peritoneal cavity. A miniature TV camera is often attached so that the surgeon, trainees, and theatre staff can see clearly. Specialized instruments are passed through other small incisions to grasp, cut, or diathermy as required. To gain a better view, carbon dioxide (CO_2) is insufflated into the peritoneal cavity and special equipment is used so that the pressure inside the peritoneum does not rise too high. Patients are intubated and ventilated for this procedure to counteract the splinting of the diaphragm and the absorption of CO_2 into the bloodstream. Things can go wrong with this technique such as overpressure of CO_2, CO_2 tracking into the chest cavity or tissues, embolism of CO_2 into blood vessels and bleeding. Sometimes, the procedure has to proceed to open operation.

The chest cavity, mediastinum, and the larger joint cavities are also suitable for endoscopic operations. The upper and lower gastrointestinal tracts can also be viewed from within using fibreoptic techniques.

Further Reading

Joris JL. Anesthetic management of laparoscopy. In: Anesthesia. 4th edition. Edited by RD Miller. Churchill Livingstone, New York. 1994. p. 2011–29.

32. Anaesthesia in the Isolated Location

N. S. Morton

Anaesthesia or anaesthetist-monitored sedation is often carried out in areas of the hospital which are isolated from the main operating theatre complex e.g. radiology department, CT scanner, MRI scanner, cardiac catheterization laboratory, radiotherapy suite, or the psychiatric unit (electroconvulsive therapy).

The principles are the same in all these areas: there must be adequate supplies of oxygen, suction equipment, anaesthesia equipment and drugs, monitoring as for all general anaesthetics, emergency drugs and equipment and defibrillator. For safety reasons there should be no compromise in these standards. Special problems include difficulty getting near to the patient, (e.g. in a scanner), adaptations of equipment for safety (e.g. non-magnetic equipment in MRI), allergic reactions to X-ray dyes (e.g. must be prepared to treat anaphylactic shock) and radiation protection of staff with lead aprons, thyroid protection collars and goggles. It is essential that staff are well trained in assisting the anaesthetist and in resuscitation procedures. Many units now insist that a senior anaesthetist be present throughout and junior trainees should not be conducting anaesthesia or sedation on their own in such isolated sites.

Further Reading

Messick JM, MacKenzie RA, Southorn P. Anesthesia at remote locations. In: Anesthesia. 4th edition. Edited by RD Miller. Churchill Livingstone, New York. 1994.

33. ORTHOPAEDICS AND TRAUMA

N. S. Morton

A wide range of general anaesthesia and local or regional anaesthesia techniques is used in orthopaedic and trauma surgery. Some patients with bone and joint disease present particular problems, such as difficult intubation (e.g. rheumatoid arthritis; ankylosing spondylitis). Positioning of patients is particularly important in orthopaedics with care required to avoid pain, stretching of nerves, dislocation of joints, movement of fractures and pressure point damage. Careful monitoring of blood loss and replacement is needed, especially for re-operation for joint replacement surgery and for spinal fusion cases. Some artificial joints are secured in place using acrylic cement and this can occasionally cause an increase or decrease in blood pressure.

Limb tourniquets are commonly used in orthopaedic surgery to reduce bleeding and to improve the surgical operating field. These comprise an air filled cuff which is inflated above the arterial blood pressure after the limb is exsanguinated by elevating it or using a rubber bandage. The tourniquet width must be correct for the size of limb (the surgeon will decide this) to avoid excess pressure on tissues under the cuff. The cuff must be carefully applied over soft padding and inflated to a pressure requested by the surgeon. The time of inflation should be noted as periods over 90–120 min may give problems with washout of lactic acid from the limb. This is because cells in the limb continue to metabolize and produce waste products. These can cause a fall in blood pressure if they suddenly enter the circulation when the tourniquet is deflated. Nerve damage in the limb can also occur with prolonged inflation times.

Another problem seen in orthopaedics and trauma is the syndrome of fat embolism where bone marrow elements get into the circulation and set off an inflammatory response. This can cause circulatory collapse and respiratory failure.

Orthopaedic patients are at particular risk of the formation of clots in the leg veins (deep venous thrombosis). These clots may detach and obstruct the lung circulation (pulmonary embolism) which can be fatal. Anticoagulants, such as heparin, are often given to present this happening and the newer forms of heparin often lessens the risk of bleeding at the time of surgery.

Trauma surgery can be particularly challenging for the anaesthetist. The anaesthetist and assistant may have to deal simultaneously with stabilizing, resuscitating and anaesthetizing a patient who may have an unstable neck, a head injury, facial injuries, chest trauma with pneumothorax or haemothorax, injury to abdominal organs such as liver, spleen, kidneys or gut and limb and pelvic fractures. The principles of basic and advanced life support apply with particular care to maintain a neutral neck position throughout. All the techniques mentioned in this book may come into play with such cases.

Further Reading

Sharrock NE, Savarese JJ. Anesthesia for orthopaedic surgery. In: Anesthesia. 4th edition. Edited by RD Miller. Churchill Livingstone, New York. 1994. p. 2125–42.

Stene JK, Grande CM. Anesthesia for trauma. In: Anesthesia. 4th edition. Edited by RD Miller. Churchill Livingstone, New York. 1994. p. 2157–73.

34. GENITOURINARY SURGERY

N. S. Morton

Patients with renal failure presenting for surgery raise particular problems. Patients are often anaemic and may have significant abnormalities of their body chemistry and fluid compartments. Particular care is required in the patient in renal failure presenting for a surgical procedure to establish vascular access for dialysis as these patients may be in cardiac failure from fluid overload and may have a high serum potassium which predisposes to abnormal heart rhythms. Many drugs used in anaesthesia are excreted from the body via the kidneys and so care is needed with doses of agents such as muscle relaxants and opioids, particularly if given in repeated doses. New agents such as atracurium and remifentanil do not rely on the kidneys for elimination and are the best for such cases as they are short acting and do not accumulate.

Many urological procedures are diagnostic endoscopic procedures to look at the bladder, urethra, and ureters. Many procedures can be performed via the endoscope (cystoscope) such as resection of bladder tumours or of the prostate gland. Whenever cystoscopies are done, the bladder is filled up with an irrigating solution containing glycine. This gives the surgeon a better view by distending the bladder and by washing away blood. After prolonged procedures this solution can be absorbed into the patient's circulation leading to fluid overload with heart failure and cerebral oedema. Other problems sometimes seen are septicaemia or endotoxin absorption from the urinary tract, perforation of the bladder, excessive bleeding, and coagulation failure.

Further Reading

Malhotra V. Anesthesia and the renal and genitourinary systems. In: Anesthesia. 4th edition. Edited by RD Miller. Churchill Livingstone, New York, 1994. pp. 1947–67.

35. TRANSPLANTATION

N. S. Morton

Transplantation surgery is a highly specialized field where advances are limited by the shortage of donor organs. Organs for transplantation are usually preserved by being filled with a special fluid solution while being cooled. This reduces the cell metabolism and preserves the cell function. Kidneys can be preserved for up to 48 hours, the liver for up to 24 hours, lungs for about 8 hours and the heart for 4 to 6 hours. Organs are obtained from certified brain dead patients after consent has been obtained from relatives. The donor operation can be upsetting to theatre staff but, although the patient is certified as brain dead, they are afforded the same care and respect given to all patients.

The transplant operation demands meticulous monitoring and excellent vascular access in patients who are often extremely ill with organ failure. Fluid and blood product requirements may be large and patients will often need intensive care support of several systems in the operating room and afterwards.

Further Reading

Firestone L, Firestone S. Organ transplantation. In: Anesthesia. 4th edition. Edited by RD Miller. Churchill Livingstone, New York. 1994. pp. 1981–2009.

36. CHRONIC PAIN

N. S. Morton

Chronic pain problems are complex and patients are best cared for by a multidisciplinary pain clinic team involving anaesthesia, neurosurgery, psychiatry, psychology, physiotherapy, oncology, and others. The key to chronic pain management is accurate diagnosis and the assessment process can be prolonged. The anaesthetist may require assistance with diagnostic or therapeutic nerve blocks and sometimes these need to be carried out in the X-ray department to ensure correct needle placement. As well as blocks of peripheral nerves and plexuses, sympathetic nervous system blocks may be used (e.g. cervical sympathetic or stellate block, lumbar sympathetic block). Coeliac plexus block is used to control the pain for example from pancreatic cancer. Epidural or spinal injection of steroids is sometimes used. In cancer, sometimes nerves are deliberately destroyed by injecting concentrated solutions of alcohol or phenol.

Further Reading

Murphy TM. Chronic pain. In: Anesthesia. 4th edition. Edited by RD Miller. Churchill Livingstone, New York. 1994. pp. 2345–73.

INDEX